The FODMAP Diet and Stress Management

A guide to managing stress and reducing inflammation on the FODMAP Diet.

TABLE OF CONTENTS

The role of physical activity in reducing inflammation and managing stress.

Lifestyle changes

Guidance on meal planning, including FODMAP-friendly foods and portion control

INTRODUCTION

In the whirlwind of our modern lives, where deadlines loom large, responsibilities seem never-ending, and the constant hum of technology is an ever-present backdrop, stress and inflammation have become all too familiar companions. Both are intricate and interconnected physiological responses with profound effects on our well-being. However, when one embarks on the challenging journey of adhering to a FODMAP diet, the significance of managing stress and inflammation is heightened to a critical level.

The FODMAP diet, short for Fermentable Oligosaccharides, Disaccharides, Monosaccharides, and Polyols, is not merely a dietary choice; it's a therapeutic approach primarily designed to alleviate the debilitating symptoms of irritable bowel syndrome (IBS) and other gastrointestinal disorders. This diet restricts the intake of specific carbohydrates and sugar alcohols, which are known to trigger digestive distress, bloating, and discomfort in those with sensitive guts.

While the FODMAP diet can offer relief from these chronic gastrointestinal problems, it's not without its own set of challenges. It necessitates careful food selection, portion control, and ongoing vigilance in identifying and avoiding FODMAP-rich ingredients. Furthermore, it's not uncommon for individuals on this diet to experience heightened stress levels related to the restrictive nature of their eating habits, concerns about social situations, and the overall management of their condition.

This is where stress management becomes indispensable. Stress, whether caused by the demands of daily life or anxiety surrounding one's dietary restrictions, can have a significant impact on gastrointestinal health. When stress hormones flood the body, it can disrupt digestion, exacerbate symptoms, and even make it more challenging to adhere to the FODMAP diet. Additionally, stress can exacerbate another critical factor in the equation: inflammation.

Inflammation, though primarily associated with injuries and infections, plays a subtler but equally vital role in the context of dietary health. Chronic inflammation is increasingly recognized as a risk factor for various health issues, including heart disease, diabetes, and autoimmune conditions. For individuals on a FODMAP diet, keeping inflammation in check is of paramount importance. This is because the gut, often referred to as the "second brain," is a hub of immune activity and inflammation regulation. Any imbalance in the gut, whether due to a dietary shift or chronic stress, can lead to systemic inflammation and worsen gastrointestinal symptoms.

Hence, this intricate web of connections between stress, inflammation, and the FODMAP diet brings us to a pivotal crossroads. In this complex journey to better gut health, it is imperative to explore strategies for managing stress and reducing inflammation. Doing so not only enhances one's overall well-being but also ensures the effectiveness of the FODMAP diet in providing relief from IBS and similar disorders. In the following discussion, we will delve into these aspects in greater detail, exploring the science behind stress and inflammation, and discovering practical, holistic approaches to manage them effectively while navigating the FODMAP diet.

PART ONE

WHAT ARE FODMAPS?

FODMAPs, an acronym for Fermentable Oligosaccharides, Disaccharides, Monosaccharides, and Polyols, are a group of short-chain carbohydrates and sugar alcohols that are poorly absorbed in the small intestine. They are known for their ability to trigger digestive symptoms, particularly in individuals with irritable bowel syndrome (IBS) and certain other gastrointestinal conditions. Here's a breakdown of what each component of the acronym represents:

• Fermentable: FODMAPs are carbohydrates that can be fermented by bacteria in the gut. When bacteria ferment these compounds, they produce gases and other byproducts, which can lead to digestive discomfort.

• Oligosaccharides: This refers to a group of carbohydrates that includes fructans and galacto-oligosaccharides. Common food sources of oligosaccharides include wheat, onions, garlic, and legumes.

• Disaccharides: These are double sugar molecules. The disaccharide of particular concern in the context of FODMAPs is lactose, found in dairy products like milk, yogurt, and soft cheeses.

• Monosaccharides: Monosaccharides are single sugar molecules. In the context of FODMAPs, the focus is primarily on excess fructose, which can be an issue in foods like honey, apples, and pears.

• Polyols: Polyols are sugar alcohols often used as artificial sweeteners. Common polyols include sorbitol, mannitol, xylitol, and maltitol. They are found naturally in some fruits like stone fruits (e.g., cherries, plums) and artificial sweeteners.

People with IBS or other digestive issues may experience gas, bloating, abdominal pain, and diarrhea when they consume foods high in FODMAPs because these carbohydrates are not well absorbed in the small intestine. The goal of a low FODMAP diet is to reduce the intake of these poorly absorbed carbohydrates to alleviate these symptoms. However, it's important to note that the FODMAP diet is typically undertaken under the guidance of a healthcare professional or a registered dietitian, as it can be restrictive and complex to follow. It's not intended for long-term use but rather as a diagnostic and short-term management tool for individuals with specific digestive conditions.

WHY SOME INDIVIDUALS FOLLOW THE FODMAP DIET?

Individuals may choose to follow the FODMAP diet for a variety of reasons, most commonly to manage digestive issues and improve their overall well-being. Here are some of the primary reasons why people opt for the FODMAP diet:

• Irritable Bowel Syndrome (IBS): The most common reason for following the FODMAP diet is to manage the symptoms of IBS, a chronic gastrointestinal disorder. FODMAPs are known to trigger symptoms such as bloating, abdominal pain, diarrhea, and constipation in people with IBS. By reducing FODMAP intake, many individuals can experience significant symptom relief.

• Digestive Discomfort: Even without a formal diagnosis of IBS, some people experience digestive discomfort, such as gas and bloating, after consuming high-FODMAP foods. These individuals may find relief by reducing their FODMAP intake.

• Inflammatory Bowel Disease (IBD): Some individuals with Crohn's disease or ulcerative colitis, both of which are forms of IBD, find that certain high-FODMAP foods exacerbate their symptoms during a flare-up. They may temporarily adopt a low-FODMAP diet to alleviate discomfort.

• Food Allergies and Sensitivities: People with known or suspected food allergies or sensitivities may use the FODMAP diet to identify specific triggers. By eliminating high-FODMAP foods and reintroducing them methodically, they can pinpoint the sources of their adverse reactions.

• Chronic Fatigue and Discomfort: There is evidence to suggest that reducing FODMAPs might help with chronic fatigue and discomfort in some individuals, even in the absence of a specific diagnosis. Such individuals may experiment with the diet to gauge its impact on their well-being.

• Improved Digestive Health: Some individuals follow the FODMAP diet as part of a broader effort to optimize their digestive health and reduce overall inflammation. A reduction in FODMAPs may lead to less gas, bloating, and digestive discomfort.

• Weight Management: In certain cases, individuals may adopt a low-FODMAP diet for weight management purposes. By reducing high-FODMAP foods that are often calorie-dense and opting for lower-FODMAP, healthier alternatives, they may be able to better manage their weight.

• Personal Experimentation: Some people may embark on a FODMAP diet out of curiosity or as a self-experiment to see if it positively impacts their well-being, even if they do not have a specific medical condition driving their choice.

It's important to note that the FODMAP diet is not a one-size-fits-all solution, and it is not intended for long-term use. It is a diagnostic and short-term management tool under the guidance of a healthcare professional or a registered dietitian. Moreover, the diet can be restrictive, so it should be undertaken with proper knowledge and support to ensure nutritional adequacy and prevent unintended consequences.

WHAT IS IBS?

Irritable Bowel Syndrome (IBS) is a common gastrointestinal disorder characterized by a range of symptoms related to the digestive system. It is a chronic condition that can cause significant discomfort and affect a person's quality of life. The exact cause of IBS is not fully understood, and it is considered a functional gastrointestinal disorder, meaning there are no structural or physical abnormalities that explain the symptoms. Instead, it is a disorder of how the digestive system functions.

Key characteristics of IBS include:

• Abdominal Pain and Discomfort: People with IBS often experience abdominal pain or discomfort, which can range from mild to severe. The pain is typically relieved by having a bowel movement.

• Changes in Bowel Habits: IBS can cause alterations in bowel habits, leading to diarrhea, constipation, or a combination of both. These changes can occur over time or may alternate between periods of diarrhea and constipation.

• Bloating and Gas: Many individuals with IBS report frequent bloating and increased gas production.

• Altered Stool Consistency: Stools may vary in consistency, from loose and watery to hard and lumpy. Some people may also experience mucus in their stools.

• Relief with Bowel Movements: IBS symptoms are often relieved or improved after a bowel movement.

• Mucus in Stools: Some individuals with IBS may notice mucus in their stools.

• Sensitivity to Food: Certain foods and dietary triggers can exacerbate IBS symptoms, and food sensitivities are common among people with IBS.

• Flare-Ups and Remissions: Symptoms of IBS can come and go, with periods of relative relief (remissions) followed by episodes of more severe symptoms (flare-ups).

It's important to note that IBS is a diagnosis of exclusion, meaning other potential causes of gastrointestinal symptoms, such as inflammatory bowel disease (IBD), celiac disease, or colon cancer, must be ruled out before IBS is diagnosed.

The specific cause of IBS remains uncertain, but various factors are believed to contribute, including abnormalities in the gut-brain axis, gut motility, and sensitivity to pain. Psychological factors, such as stress and anxiety, can also play a role in triggering or exacerbating IBS symptoms.

IBS can be managed and treated through dietary modifications, lifestyle changes, stress management, and, in some cases, medications prescribed by a healthcare professional. If you suspect you have IBS or are experiencing persistent gastrointestinal symptoms, it is crucial to consult with a healthcare provider for a proper diagnosis and guidance on managing the condition.

HOW TO MANAGE IBS

Managing irritable bowel syndrome (IBS) involves a multifaceted approach that combines dietary modifications, lifestyle changes, stress management, and potential medical interventions. Here's a step-by-step guide on how to manage IBS:

1. Seek a Medical Diagnosis:

If you suspect you have IBS or are experiencing persistent gastrointestinal symptoms such as abdominal pain, bloating, diarrhea, or constipation, consult a healthcare professional. They can diagnose IBS and rule out other potential underlying conditions.

2. Understand Your Triggers:

Keep a detailed food and symptom diary to identify specific foods or situations that trigger your IBS symptoms. Understanding your triggers is a crucial step in managing IBS.

3. Consult with a Healthcare Professional:

Work with a healthcare professional, such as a gastroenterologist or a registered dietitian, who specializes in gastrointestinal disorders. They can provide personalized guidance and treatment options tailored to your needs.

4. Dietary Modifications:

Consider implementing a low-FODMAP diet, which restricts certain types of carbohydrates that can trigger IBS symptoms. This diet has three phases: elimination, reintroduction, and maintenance. Consult a registered dietitian for guidance on this diet.

5. Fiber Management:

Adjust your fiber intake to alleviate symptoms. Soluble fiber can help with diarrhea, while insoluble fiber may be better for constipation. Foods like oats, flaxseeds, and psyllium husk can provide soluble fiber.

6. Hydration:

Stay well-hydrated to support digestive health and prevent dehydration associated with diarrhea.

7. Small, Frequent Meals:

Instead of large meals, consider eating smaller, more frequent meals to reduce the load on your digestive system and minimize symptoms.

8. Probiotics:

Discuss the use of probiotics with your healthcare provider. They can recommend specific strains that might help regulate gut bacteria and reduce IBS symptoms.

9. Stress Management:

Practice stress-reduction techniques like mindfulness, meditation, deep breathing, or yoga to manage emotional stress, which can trigger IBS symptoms.

10. Regular Exercise:

Engage in regular physical activity to promote overall well-being and help manage IBS. Exercise can reduce stress, improve digestion, and relieve constipation.

11. Medications:

If dietary and lifestyle changes alone do not effectively manage your IBS symptoms, your healthcare provider may prescribe medications. These can include antispasmodic drugs, laxatives, antidiarrheal medications, or medications to manage pain or anxiety.

12. Evaluate Your Trigger Foods:

After the elimination phase of the low-FODMAP diet, you can gradually reintroduce specific FODMAP groups to identify your personal triggers. This will help you create a more personalized dietary plan.

13. Monitor Your Symptoms:

Continue to track your symptoms and dietary habits to assess your progress. This can help you make necessary adjustments.

14. Be Patient:

Managing IBS is a gradual process, and it may take some time to find the right combination of dietary and lifestyle changes that work for you. Be patient and persistent in your efforts.

15. Regular Check-Ins:

Maintain regular check-ins with your healthcare provider or dietitian to discuss your progress, make necessary modifications to your plan, and ensure your IBS is well-managed.

Remember that IBS management is highly individual, and what works for one person may not work for another. It's important to work closely with healthcare professionals to develop a customized plan tailored to your specific needs and preferences.

AN OVERVIEW OF WHAT STRESS AND INFLAMMATION ARE AND HOW THEY CAN IMPACT OVERALL HEALTH

1. Stress:

Stress is the body's natural response to various challenges and demands, whether they are physical, emotional, or psychological. It is a normal and often necessary part of life, helping us cope with situations that require alertness and action. However, chronic or excessive stress can have significant negative impacts on overall health.

• Acute vs. Chronic Stress: Acute stress is short-term and often motivates us to solve problems or respond to immediate threats (the "fight or flight" response). Chronic stress, on the other hand, is persistent and long-lasting, and it can lead to health issues when the body's stress response is constantly activated.

• Effects of Stress on Health: Chronic stress can contribute to a wide range of health problems, including high blood pressure, cardiovascular disease, digestive disorders, weakened immune function, anxiety, depression, and sleep disturbances. It can also exacerbate existing health conditions and decrease overall well-being.

2. Inflammation:

Inflammation is the body's natural response to injury, infection, or irritation. It is a protective mechanism aimed at removing harmful stimuli and initiating the healing process. There are two types of inflammation:

• Acute Inflammation: This is a short-term response to an injury or infection and is generally beneficial. It involves the release of inflammatory molecules and the activation of immune cells to address the issue and promote healing.

• Chronic Inflammation: Unlike acute inflammation, chronic inflammation is long-term and can be harmful. It occurs when the body's inflammatory response is activated over an extended period, often without a clear threat to address. Chronic inflammation is associated with many health conditions, including cardiovascular disease, autoimmune disorders, obesity, and cancer.

3. How Stress and Inflammation Are Interrelated and Impact Health:

Stress and inflammation are closely connected, and one can influence the other. Stress can trigger the release of stress hormones like cortisol, which can lead to increased levels of inflammation in the body. This relationship has significant implications for overall health:

• Impact on Immune System: Chronic stress and inflammation can weaken the immune system, making the body more susceptible to infections and impairing its ability to defend against diseases.

• Cardiovascular Health: Chronic inflammation is a key driver of atherosclerosis, which is a process that can lead to heart disease. Stress, especially chronic stress, can contribute to hypertension and other cardiovascular risk factors.

• Mental Health: Chronic inflammation is also associated with mental health issues, including depression and anxiety. In turn, experiencing chronic stress can contribute to these mental health conditions.

• Digestive Health: Inflammation in the gastrointestinal tract can be exacerbated by stress, potentially leading to digestive disorders, such as irritable bowel syndrome (IBS).

• Chronic Diseases: Chronic stress and inflammation are implicated in the development and exacerbation of chronic diseases, including autoimmune diseases and certain types of cancer.

Managing and mitigating stress through stress-reduction techniques such as relaxation, mindfulness, and exercise can help reduce inflammation and its associated health risks. Similarly, adopting a healthy lifestyle, including a balanced diet and regular physical activity, can help regulate the body's inflammatory response and promote overall health and well-being.

THE CONNECTION BETWEEN STRESS, INFLAMMATION AND DIGESTIVE HEALTH

The connection between stress, inflammation, and digestive health is a complex and bidirectional relationship. Stress can impact digestive health, and digestive issues can, in turn, cause or exacerbate stress. Here's a closer look at this interplay:

1. Stress and Digestive Health:

• Stress Response: When the body encounters a stressful situation, it activates the "fight or flight" response, releasing stress hormones like cortisol. This response diverts resources away from functions like digestion and immune response.

• Slowed Digestion: Stress can lead to slowed digestion, as the body prioritizes immediate survival over long-term processes. This can result in symptoms like abdominal discomfort, bloating, and changes in bowel habits.

• Gut-Brain Axis: There is a strong connection between the brain and the gut, known as the gut-brain axis. Stress can affect this communication system, leading to changes in gut motility, sensitivity, and function. Stress can also influence gut bacteria composition.

• Exacerbation of Digestive Conditions: For individuals with preexisting digestive conditions like irritable bowel syndrome (IBS), inflammatory bowel disease (IBD), or gastroesophageal reflux disease (GERD), stress can exacerbate symptoms and trigger flare-ups.

2. Inflammation and Digestive Health:

• Inflammatory Response: Inflammation is a natural response to injury or infection in the body. However, chronic inflammation in the gastrointestinal tract can be harmful and is associated with conditions like Crohn's disease, ulcerative colitis, and celiac disease.

• Digestive Disorders: Inflammation can contribute to the development and progression of various digestive disorders. For example, in IBD, the immune system mistakenly attacks the digestive tract, leading to chronic inflammation and symptoms like abdominal pain and diarrhea.

• Chronic Stress and Inflammation: Chronic stress can lead to a state of chronic low-grade inflammation throughout the body. This inflammation can extend to the gastrointestinal system, potentially contributing to the development or worsening of digestive conditions.

3. The Bidirectional Relationship:

• Vicious Cycle: Stress can trigger or exacerbate digestive issues, which, in turn, can cause stress due to the discomfort and unpredictability of symptoms. This creates a vicious cycle, where stress and digestive symptoms continually feed into each other.

• Mind-Body Connection: The connection between stress, inflammation, and digestive health highlights the importance of the mind-body connection. Emotional stress can manifest physically in the gut, leading to digestive symptoms. Similarly, chronic inflammation in the gut can signal the brain and lead to feelings of stress or anxiety.

4. Managing this complex relationship involves:

• Stress Management: Practicing stress-reduction techniques like mindfulness, relaxation, deep breathing, and regular physical activity can help reduce the impact of stress on digestive health.

• Dietary Choices: Following a balanced diet, including foods that support gut health (e.g., fiber, probiotics), and identifying and avoiding trigger foods (e.g., high-FODMAP foods for some individuals) can be crucial for managing digestive conditions.

• Medical Care: Seeking medical care from a healthcare provider or gastroenterologist is essential for the diagnosis and management of digestive conditions and chronic inflammation.

• Medications: In some cases, medications may be prescribed to manage inflammation and digestive symptoms.

Understanding and addressing the connections between stress, inflammation, and digestive health is vital for comprehensive gastrointestinal care and overall well-being.

UNDERSTANDING INFLAMMATION AND ITS RELATIONSHIP WITH DIET

Inflammation is a fundamental biological response that occurs in the body as a defense mechanism against various threats, including infections, injuries, and irritants. While acute inflammation is a necessary and beneficial part of the body's immune response, chronic inflammation can be harmful and is linked to various health conditions. The relationship between inflammation and diet is significant, as the foods we consume can either promote or mitigate inflammation in the body.

Here is an overview of inflammation and its relationship with diet:

1. Types of Inflammation:

• Acute Inflammation: This is a short-term response to an immediate threat, such as an infection or injury. It involves the activation of immune cells and the release of inflammatory molecules to address the issue. Acute inflammation is a necessary part of the healing process.

• Chronic Inflammation: Chronic inflammation is a long-lasting, low-grade, and often systemic response. It can result from various factors, including persistent infections, autoimmune disorders, and lifestyle factors, such as poor diet. Chronic inflammation is linked to a range of health conditions, including heart disease, type 2 diabetes, certain cancers, and neurodegenerative diseases.

2. Diet and Inflammation:

• Pro-Inflammatory Foods: Some foods are known to promote inflammation in the body. These typically include highly processed and sugary foods, trans fats, and those high in saturated fats. Sugary drinks, refined carbohydrates, and red meat are examples of pro-inflammatory foods.

• Anti-Inflammatory Foods: Conversely, certain foods have anti-inflammatory properties and can help reduce inflammation in the body. These include fruits, vegetables, whole grains, fatty fish rich in omega-3 fatty acids (e.g., salmon, mackerel), nuts, seeds, and herbs like turmeric and ginger.

These foods are rich in antioxidants, which can help counteract the effects of inflammation.

3. Dietary Patterns:

• Mediterranean Diet: The Mediterranean diet, rich in fruits, vegetables, whole grains, and healthy fats (olive oil, nuts), is often associated with reduced inflammation and a lower risk of chronic diseases.

• Anti-Inflammatory Diet: Some individuals follow an anti-inflammatory diet, which emphasizes foods known for their anti-inflammatory properties. It typically includes a wide variety of fruits, vegetables, whole grains, lean proteins, and fatty fish.

4. Weight and Inflammation:

Excess body fat, especially abdominal obesity, is associated with higher levels of inflammation. Losing weight through a combination of a balanced diet and regular physical activity can reduce inflammation in the body.

5. Individual Variation:

The relationship between diet and inflammation can vary among individuals. Genetics, lifestyle factors, and preexisting health conditions all play a role in determining how specific foods affect a person's inflammation levels.

6. Specialized Diets:

Some individuals with chronic conditions associated with inflammation, such as rheumatoid arthritis or inflammatory bowel disease, may benefit from specialized dietary approaches designed to reduce inflammation and manage their symptoms.

In summary, the foods we eat have a significant impact on inflammation in the body. A diet rich in anti-inflammatory foods and low in pro-inflammatory foods is associated with reduced chronic inflammation and a lower risk of inflammatory-related diseases. When considering dietary changes to reduce inflammation, it's essential to consult with a healthcare professional or registered dietitian to create a well-balanced, personalized eating plan that aligns with individual health goals and needs.

THE FODMAP DIET, INCLUDING WHAT IT ENTAILS AND WHO IT IS DESIGNED FOR

The FODMAP diet, which stands for Fermentable Oligosaccharides, Disaccharides, Monosaccharides, and Polyols, is a dietary approach designed to manage symptoms associated with certain gastrointestinal conditions, primarily irritable bowel syndrome (IBS). Here's an overview of what the FODMAP diet entails and who it is designed for:

What the FODMAP Diet Entails:

The FODMAP diet is a structured dietary plan that focuses on reducing the intake of specific types of fermentable carbohydrates and sugar alcohols, known as FODMAPs, which are poorly absorbed in the small intestine. These substances can ferment in the colon, leading to the production of gas and other byproducts that may trigger gastrointestinal symptoms such as bloating, gas, abdominal pain, and altered bowel habits in susceptible individuals.

The FODMAP diet typically consists of three main phases:

• Elimination Phase: During this phase, individuals restrict their intake of high-FODMAP foods to minimize their symptoms. Common high-FODMAP foods include certain fruits (e.g., apples, pears), vegetables (e.g., onions, garlic), dairy products, wheat-based products, and artificial sweeteners. The elimination phase usually lasts 2-6 weeks.

• Reintroduction Phase: After the elimination phase, individuals systematically reintroduce specific FODMAP groups one at a time to identify which FODMAPs trigger their symptoms. This phase helps individuals identify their personal FODMAP triggers, allowing for a more personalized diet.

• Maintenance Phase: Once trigger foods are identified, individuals can follow a modified diet that avoids only the FODMAPs that cause symptoms. The goal is to have a balanced diet that is as varied as possible, while still managing symptoms.

Who the FODMAP Diet Is Designed For:

The FODMAP diet is primarily designed for individuals who have been diagnosed with or are experiencing symptoms of irritable bowel syndrome (IBS) and related gastrointestinal conditions. IBS is a common digestive disorder characterized by abdominal pain, bloating, and altered bowel habits, often without any visible structural abnormalities in the gut.

The diet is specifically intended for individuals who experience relief from their gastrointestinal symptoms when following a low-FODMAP diet. It is not a one-size-fits-all approach, as individual tolerance to FODMAPs varies. This diet is also not intended for long-term use, as it can be restrictive and may reduce the intake of some healthy foods, such as fruits, vegetables, and whole grains.

It's essential to note that the FODMAP diet should be undertaken under the guidance of a healthcare professional or a registered dietitian. They can provide personalized recommendations, ensure nutritional adequacy, and help individuals navigate the complexities of the diet.

In summary, the FODMAP diet is a structured dietary plan designed to alleviate symptoms of IBS and related conditions by reducing the intake of specific fermentable carbohydrates. It is suitable for individuals who experience relief from their digestive symptoms when following this approach and is best managed with professional guidance.

The FODMAP diet is typically divided into three main phases: the Elimination Phase, the Reintroduction Phase, and the Maintenance Phase. These phases are designed to help individuals with digestive issues like irritable bowel syndrome (IBS) identify and manage their specific FODMAP triggers while maintaining a balanced diet. Here's an explanation of each phase:

1. Elimination Phase:

The Elimination Phase is the initial stage of the FODMAP diet and typically lasts for 2 to 6 weeks. During this phase, individuals restrict their intake of high-FODMAP foods as much as possible to minimize symptoms. The primary goal is to achieve symptom relief and create a "clean slate" before reintroducing specific FODMAPs to identify individual triggers.

Key Steps and Guidelines:

• Identify High-FODMAP Foods: Work with a registered dietitian or healthcare professional to identify foods that are high in FODMAPs. Common high-FODMAP foods include certain fruits (e.g., apples, pears), vegetables (e.g., onions, garlic), dairy products, wheat-based products, and artificial sweeteners.

• Strict Avoidance: Eliminate high-FODMAP foods from your diet, while focusing on consuming low-FODMAP alternatives. Be vigilant about food labels and ingredient lists to avoid hidden sources of FODMAPs.

• Monitor Symptoms: Keep a detailed food diary to track your symptoms and any changes during this phase. This will help gauge your progress and inform discussions with your dietitian.

2. Reintroduction Phase:

The Reintroduction Phase follows the Elimination Phase and is aimed at systematically reintroducing specific FODMAP groups, one at a time, to identify which FODMAPs trigger symptoms in your individual case.

• Select One FODMAP Group: Work with your dietitian to choose a specific FODMAP group to reintroduce. Examples include fructans, lactose, fructose, and polyols.

• Gradual Reintroduction: Gradually reintroduce small amounts of foods containing the selected FODMAP group while closely monitoring symptoms. If no symptoms occur, you can likely tolerate that particular FODMAP group.

• Record and Evaluate: Maintain a food diary during this phase to track your symptoms and identify any trigger foods. This information will help you determine which FODMAPs you can safely reintroduce.

• Repeat for Other Groups: Continue this process, systematically reintroducing different FODMAP groups, until you have identified your specific triggers. This helps you create a personalized dietary plan.

3. Maintenance Phase:

The Maintenance Phase follows the Reintroduction Phase and is focused on adopting a modified diet that avoids only the

FODMAPs that have been identified as triggers for your symptoms.

Key Steps and Guidelines:

• Personalized Diet: With the guidance of your dietitian, you will create a personalized diet that avoids only the FODMAPs that trigger your symptoms. This allows for a more balanced and varied diet while managing gastrointestinal discomfort.

• Long-Term Approach: The goal is to maintain this modified diet for the long term, but it should be nutritionally balanced and diverse to ensure you are getting all the necessary nutrients.

• Regular Monitoring: Continue monitoring your symptoms and adjusting your diet as needed to maintain digestive comfort. Periodic check-ins with your dietitian may be beneficial.

The FODMAP diet should be undertaken under the guidance of a healthcare professional or registered dietitian, as it can be complex and restrictive. The diet is not intended for long-term use but rather as a diagnostic and short-term management tool for individuals with specific digestive conditions.

Stress management techniques are strategies and practices aimed at reducing or coping with stress to promote mental and physical well-being. Stress is a common part of life, but chronic or excessive stress can lead to various health issues. Employing effective stress management techniques can help individuals better handle stress and improve their overall quality of life. Here are some stress management techniques:

1. Mindfulness Meditation:

Mindfulness meditation involves focusing on the present moment and accepting it without judgment. It helps reduce stress by calming the mind, promoting relaxation, and improving emotional regulation.

2. Deep Breathing:

Deep breathing exercises, like diaphragmatic or abdominal breathing, help calm the body's stress response. By taking slow, deep breaths, individuals can reduce tension and anxiety.

3. Progressive Muscle Relaxation:

This technique involves systematically tensing and relaxing different muscle groups. It can help release physical tension and promote a sense of calm.

4. Yoga:

Yoga combines physical postures, breathing exercises, and meditation to reduce stress, improve flexibility, and enhance overall well-being.

5. Exercise:

Regular physical activity, such as walking, jogging, or cycling, releases endorphins, the body's natural stress relievers. Exercise also helps improve sleep and overall mood.

6. Time Management:

Effective time management techniques, such as setting goals, prioritizing tasks, and creating a schedule, can help reduce stress related to feeling overwhelmed or rushed.

7. Social Support:

Talking to friends, family, or a therapist can provide emotional support and a healthy outlet for stress. Social connections and a support network are important for coping with stress.

8. Problem-Solving:

Identifying the source of stress and developing practical solutions can help individuals regain a sense of control and reduce stress related to specific issues.

9. Relaxation Techniques:

Activities like taking a warm bath, listening to calming music, or engaging in hobbies can promote relaxation and alleviate stress.

10. Cognitive-Behavioral Techniques:

Cognitive-behavioral therapy (CBT) can help individuals recognize and challenge negative thought patterns, reframe stressful situations, and develop healthier coping strategies.

11. Journaling:

Keeping a journal to express thoughts and feelings can be therapeutic and help individuals gain insights into sources of stress.

12. Biofeedback:

Biofeedback techniques use sensors to monitor physiological responses (e.g., heart rate or muscle tension) and teach individuals to control these responses, which can reduce stress.

13. Sleep Hygiene:

Getting sufficient, quality sleep is crucial for stress management. Establishing a regular sleep schedule and creating a relaxing bedtime routine can promote better sleep.

14. Dietary and Lifestyle Choices:

Eating a balanced diet, reducing caffeine and alcohol intake, and avoiding excessive sugar can help stabilize mood and energy levels, which in turn can reduce stress. Regular physical activity and avoiding tobacco also contribute to overall stress reduction.

15. Time for Self-Care:

Setting aside time for self-care activities, such as reading, taking a bath, or practicing a hobby, can provide relaxation and serve as a buffer against stress.

Individuals should experiment with different stress management techniques to determine what works best for them, as the effectiveness of these techniques can vary from person to person. Combining several strategies and seeking professional help when needed can be especially effective for managing stress and improving overall mental and physical health.

PRACTICAL TIPS AND STRATEGIES FOR MANAGING STRESS AND INFLAMMATION THROUGH DIET AND LIFESTYLE CHANGES.

Managing stress and inflammation through diet and lifestyle changes is crucial for overall health and well-being. Here are practical tips and strategies to help you reduce stress and inflammation:

• Regular Physical Activity: Engage in regular exercise, such as walking, jogging, yoga, or dancing. Exercise releases endorphins, which are natural stress relievers.

• Mindfulness and Meditation: Practice mindfulness meditation or deep-breathing exercises to calm the mind and reduce stress. These techniques can be integrated into your daily routine.

• Time Management: Prioritize tasks, set achievable goals, and create a daily schedule to reduce stress related to feeling overwhelmed or rushed.

• Social Support: Connect with friends and family. Talking to loved ones or a therapist can provide emotional support and a healthy outlet for stress.

• Quality Sleep: Establish a regular sleep schedule and create a relaxing bedtime routine. Getting enough rest is crucial for stress management.

• Limit Caffeine and Alcohol: Reduce caffeine and alcohol consumption, as they can contribute to stress and disrupt sleep patterns.

Inflammation Management:

• Anti-Inflammatory Diet: Focus on a diet rich in anti-inflammatory foods, including fruits, vegetables, whole grains, fatty fish (e.g., salmon), nuts, and seeds. Incorporate herbs and spices like turmeric and ginger.

• Omega-3 Fatty Acids: Increase your intake of foods high in omega-3 fatty acids, such as flaxseeds, chia seeds, walnuts, and fatty fish. Omega-3s have anti-inflammatory properties.

• Limit Saturated and Trans Fats: Reduce consumption of saturated and trans fats found in processed and fried foods. Choose healthier cooking oils like olive oil or avocado oil.

• Fiber-Rich Foods: Include plenty of fiber from whole grains, fruits, and vegetables in your diet. Fiber helps reduce inflammation and supports a healthy gut.

• Probiotics: Consume probiotic-rich foods like yogurt and kefir to support a healthy gut microbiome. A balanced gut can help manage inflammation.

• Antioxidants: Eat foods rich in antioxidants, such as berries, leafy greens, and nuts, to combat oxidative stress and inflammation.

Lifestyle Changes:

• Stress Reduction: Engage in stress-reduction techniques like mindfulness, relaxation, and deep breathing to lower chronic stress and its associated inflammation.

• Regular Exercise: Maintain a regular exercise routine to promote overall health and reduce inflammation.

• Weight Management: Achieving and maintaining a healthy weight can help reduce inflammation, especially if you have excess body fat.

• Hydration: Drink plenty of water to support overall health and reduce inflammation.

• Smoking Cessation: Quit smoking, as it is a significant source of inflammation and contributes to various health issues.

• Alcohol Moderation: Limit alcohol consumption to reduce inflammation and minimize its impact on overall health.

• Sleep Hygiene: Prioritize sleep and establish a sleep routine to support your body's natural healing processes.

Remember that stress and inflammation management is an ongoing process, and individual responses can vary. It's essential to work with healthcare professionals or registered dietitians to develop a personalized plan that aligns with your specific needs and goals. Making these lifestyle and dietary changes can significantly improve your overall health and reduce the impact of stress and inflammation on your well-being.

STEP-BY-STEP INSTRUCTIONS FOR IMPLEMENTING THE FODMAP DIET AND STRESS-REDUCTION TECHNIQUES.

Implementing the FODMAP diet and stress-reduction techniques involves a structured approach to dietary changes and mindfulness practices. Here are step-by-step instructions for each:

Implementing the FODMAP Diet:

It's important to consult with a healthcare professional or a registered dietitian before starting the FODMAP diet to ensure that it's appropriate for your specific needs.

Step 1: Consultation with a Healthcare Professional:

Schedule an appointment with a healthcare professional or registered dietitian who specializes in the FODMAP diet or gastrointestinal conditions like IBS. Discuss your symptoms, medical history, and dietary habits.

Step 2: Assessment and Diagnosis:

Work with your healthcare provider to diagnose any underlying gastrointestinal conditions, such as IBS or food intolerances, that may warrant the FODMAP diet. This may include tests and assessments.

Step 3: Education and Preparation:

Learn about the FODMAP diet and understand which foods are high and low in FODMAPs. Your healthcare provider or dietitian will provide educational materials and resources.

Step 4: Elimination Phase:

Start the FODMAP diet by eliminating high-FODMAP foods from your diet. This phase typically lasts for 2 to 6 weeks. You may need to follow a strict low-FODMAP diet during this time.

Step 5: Food Planning:

Plan your meals carefully, incorporating low-FODMAP foods and avoiding high-FODMAP sources. This may involve reading food labels and recipes to ensure compliance.

Step 6: Symptom Monitoring:

Keep a detailed food diary to monitor your symptoms throughout the Elimination Phase. Note any changes or relief in symptoms and share this information with your healthcare provider or dietitian.

Step 7: Reintroduction Phase:

Under the guidance of your healthcare provider or dietitian, systematically reintroduce specific FODMAP groups, one at a time, to identify your personal triggers. Keep a food diary during this phase to track your symptoms.

Step 8: Personalized Diet:

Once you have identified your FODMAP triggers, work with your dietitian to create a personalized diet that avoids only the specific FODMAPs that cause your symptoms.

Implementing Stress-Reduction Techniques:

Step 1: Identify Stressors:

Start by identifying the specific stressors in your life. Reflect on what causes stress and what situations or factors contribute to your overall stress levels.

Step 2: Set Realistic Goals:

Establish clear, achievable goals for stress reduction. These goals can be related to your work-life balance, relationships, or personal well-being.

Step 3: Prioritize Self-Care:

Dedicate time to self-care activities, such as mindfulness, exercise, or hobbies that bring you joy. Prioritizing self-care is essential for managing stress.

Step 4: Mindfulness and Relaxation:

Practice mindfulness meditation or deep-breathing exercises regularly to calm your mind and reduce stress. Incorporate these techniques into your daily routine.

Step 5: Time Management:

Improve your time management skills to reduce feelings of being rushed or overwhelmed. Prioritize tasks and set specific goals to make better use of your time.

Step 6: Social Support:

Connect with friends and family. Talking to loved ones or a therapist can provide emotional support and a healthy outlet for stress.

Step 7: Regular Exercise:

Engage in regular physical activity, as exercise releases endorphins, the body's natural stress relievers. Establish a consistent exercise routine.

Step 8: Maintain a Healthy Lifestyle:

Focus on a balanced diet, quality sleep, and limiting caffeine and alcohol consumption to support overall well-being and reduce stress.

Step 9: Seek Professional Help:

If stress remains unmanageable, consider seeking the help of a mental health professional or counselor who can provide specific strategies for stress reduction.

Both the FODMAP diet and stress-reduction techniques require a personalized approach. Consultation with healthcare professionals or specialists is crucial to ensure that the dietary and lifestyle changes you make are appropriate for your unique needs and circumstances.

THE ROLE OF PHYSICAL ACTIVITY IN REDUCING INFLAMMATION AND MANAGING STRESS.

Physical activity plays a significant role in reducing inflammation and managing stress, and its positive effects on both aspects of health are well-established. Here's an overview of the role of physical activity in these processes:

• Anti-Inflammatory Effects: Regular physical activity has anti-inflammatory effects on the body. It reduces the production of pro-inflammatory cytokines and increases the release of anti-inflammatory cytokines. This balanced cytokine profile can help reduce chronic inflammation, which is linked to various health conditions, including heart disease, diabetes, and autoimmune disorders.

• Weight Management: Exercise is essential for weight management, and maintaining a healthy weight is a key factor in reducing inflammation. Excess body fat, especially abdominal obesity, is associated with increased inflammation. Exercise helps to burn calories, shed excess fat, and reduce inflammation in the process.

• Insulin Sensitivity: Physical activity improves insulin sensitivity and glucose regulation. This, in turn, can help reduce inflammation, as high blood sugar levels are linked to increased inflammation.

• Enhancing Immune Function: Moderate exercise supports immune function by increasing the activity of immune cells. A well-functioning immune system can help control inflammation and protect against infections and diseases.

Managing Stress:

• Stress Hormone Regulation: Exercise helps regulate stress hormones, such as cortisol and adrenaline. Physical activity prompts the release of endorphins, which are natural mood lifters. It also reduces the production of stress hormones, which can alleviate feelings of anxiety and tension.

• Stress Reduction: Engaging in physical activity provides a healthy outlet for stress and pent-up emotions. It helps individuals release built-up tension, promoting relaxation and improved mood.

• Mind-Body Connection: Many forms of exercise, such as yoga and tai chi, emphasize the mind-body connection. These practices incorporate mindfulness and deep breathing, helping individuals become more aware of their body and reduce stress through relaxation techniques.

• Quality Sleep: Regular exercise can improve the quality of sleep. A good night's sleep is essential for stress management, as sleep helps the body recover and recharge. Sleep disturbances are often associated with increased stress levels.

• Social Interaction: Participating in group activities, team sports, or fitness classes can provide social support and a sense of community, which can be valuable for stress reduction.

Balancing Physical Activity for Stress and Inflammation:

It's important to strike a balance in physical activity. While regular exercise is beneficial for managing stress and reducing inflammation, excessive or intense exercise without adequate recovery can lead to stress and inflammation. Overtraining can have negative consequences on both physical and mental health. A well-rounded exercise program that includes aerobic activity, strength training, flexibility exercises, and relaxation techniques can provide the most comprehensive benefits for stress and inflammation management.

Before starting a new exercise program, it's advisable to consult with a healthcare provider, especially if you have underlying health conditions. They can provide guidance on the most suitable exercise routine for your individual needs and help you create a balanced plan that supports your well-being.

Lifestyle changes are essential for managing stress and inflammation, and they complement other strategies like diet and exercise. Here are some key lifestyle changes that can help reduce stress and inflammation:

1. Prioritize Quality Sleep:

• Sleep Hygiene: Establish a regular sleep schedule, aiming for 7-9 hours of quality sleep each night. Create a bedtime routine that promotes relaxation, such as reading, taking a warm bath, or practicing deep breathing exercises.

• Limit Screen Time: Reduce exposure to screens (phones, tablets, computers, TVs) before bedtime, as the blue light emitted from screens can interfere with your natural sleep-wake cycle.

• Sleep Environment: Make your bedroom conducive to sleep by keeping it cool, dark, and quiet. Invest in a comfortable mattress and pillows.

• Caffeine and Alcohol: Limit caffeine and alcohol intake, especially in the hours leading up to bedtime, as they can disrupt sleep patterns.

2. Maintain a Support Network:

• Stay Connected: Cultivate and maintain meaningful relationships with friends, family, or support groups. Social connections provide emotional support and a sense of belonging.

• Open Communication: Share your thoughts and feelings with trusted individuals. Talking about your stressors and concerns can help alleviate emotional burdens.

• Seek Professional Help: If stress becomes overwhelming, consider consulting a therapist or counselor. They can provide guidance and support for managing stress and improving emotional well-being.

3. Practice Mindfulness and Relaxation:

• Mindfulness Meditation: Incorporate mindfulness meditation or deep-breathing exercises into your daily routine. These practices help you stay present, reduce stress, and improve emotional regulation.

• Yoga and Tai Chi: Engage in activities that emphasize the mind-body connection, such as yoga and tai chi. These practices promote relaxation, flexibility, and stress reduction.

• Hobbies and Leisure Activities: Dedicate time to activities you enjoy, whether it's painting, gardening, playing a musical instrument, or any other hobby. These pursuits provide a healthy outlet for stress and foster creativity.

4. Time Management and Goal Setting:

• Set Realistic Goals: Establish clear, achievable goals for stress reduction. Break larger goals into smaller, manageable tasks to prevent feeling overwhelmed.

• Effective Time Management: Improve your time management skills by prioritizing tasks and creating a daily schedule. This can help you make better use of your time and reduce stress.

5. Maintain a Healthy Lifestyle:

• Balanced Diet: Follow a balanced, nutrient-dense diet that includes plenty of fruits, vegetables, whole grains, lean proteins, and healthy fats. A well-rounded diet supports overall health and reduces inflammation.

• Regular Physical Activity: Engage in regular exercise to reduce stress, improve mood, and manage inflammation. Incorporate a combination of aerobic, strength, and flexibility exercises into your routine.

• Stress Reduction Techniques: Explore stress management techniques like progressive muscle relaxation, biofeedback, or cognitive-behavioral therapy to identify and address sources of stress.

6. Limit Toxins and Negative Influences:

• Tobacco and Alcohol: If you smoke, seek support to quit. Limit alcohol consumption, as it can contribute to stress and inflammation.

• Avoid Excessive Sugar: Reduce your intake of processed foods and sugary snacks, as excessive sugar consumption can contribute to inflammation.

7. Mindful Communication:

Practice effective and mindful communication. Listen actively, express your thoughts clearly, and avoid negative or aggressive communication styles.

8. Time for Self-Care:

Dedicate time for self-care activities, whether it's reading, taking a warm bath, or practicing a hobby. Prioritizing self-care helps reduce stress and promotes relaxation.

Remember that lifestyle changes are most effective when incorporated into a holistic approach to well-being. It's essential to tailor these changes to your individual needs and circumstances, and consulting with healthcare professionals, therapists, or registered dietitians can provide valuable guidance and support.

GUIDANCE ON MEAL PLANNING, INCLUDING FODMAP-FRIENDLY FOODS AND PORTION CONTROL

Meal planning can be a helpful strategy for individuals following a low-FODMAP diet, as it ensures that you have a variety of FODMAP-friendly foods while controlling portion sizes. Here's guidance on meal planning for the FODMAP diet, including food choices and portion control:

1. Food Choices:

Low-FODMAP Foods: Focus on incorporating foods that are low in FODMAPs. Some examples of low-FODMAP foods include:

• Proteins: Chicken, turkey, fish, tofu, and eggs.

• Vegetables: Spinach, zucchini, carrots, bell peppers, and green beans.

• Fruits: Strawberries, blueberries, oranges, and grapes (in small portions).

• Grains: Rice (white, brown), quinoa, oats (if tolerated).

• Dairy Alternatives: Lactose-free milk, almond milk, and lactose-free yogurt.

Moderate-FODMAP Foods: Some foods are moderate in FODMAPs and may be tolerated in small quantities. These include:

• Proteins: Beef, pork, and certain seafood.

• Vegetables: Sweet potatoes, broccoli, and asparagus (in small portions).

• Fruits: Bananas, kiwi (in small portions).

• Grains: Gluten-free bread, pasta, and cereals.

2. Portion Control:

Portion control is essential, even with low-FODMAP foods. Here are some tips:

• Follow Serving Sizes: Pay attention to recommended serving sizes on food labels and use measuring cups or a kitchen scale if necessary.

• Start Small: If you're unsure about tolerating a moderate-FODMAP food, begin with a small portion and gradually increase it while monitoring your symptoms.

• Listen to Your Body: Be mindful of your body's signals. If you experience discomfort or digestive issues after a meal, it might be due to portion size, even if you're eating low-FODMAP foods.

3. Balanced Meals:

When planning your meals, aim for a balance of macronutrients (carbohydrates, protein, and fat). Here's a general structure to follow:

• Proteins: Include a source of lean protein in each meal, such as chicken, fish, tofu, or eggs.

• Vegetables: Incorporate a variety of low-FODMAP vegetables, like spinach, carrots, and bell peppers. Be mindful of portion sizes for moderate-FODMAP options.

• Grains: Opt for low-FODMAP grains like rice or quinoa, or gluten-free options if necessary.

• Fats: Include healthy fats from sources like olive oil, nuts, and seeds.

4. Snacks:

Plan low-FODMAP snacks to keep your energy levels stable between meals. Suitable options include:

• Small portions of low-FODMAP fruits like strawberries or blueberries.

• Lactose-free yogurt or lactose-free cheese.

• Rice cakes with peanut or almond butter.

• Nuts and seeds (in moderation).

- Carrot or cucumber sticks with hummus (be mindful of portion size).

5. Read Labels:

When purchasing packaged foods, read labels carefully to ensure they do not contain high-FODMAP ingredients or additives that can trigger symptoms.

6. Keep a Food Diary:

Maintain a food diary to track your meals, portion sizes, and symptoms. This can help you identify which foods and portion sizes work best for your individual tolerance.

7. Consult a Dietitian:

Working with a registered dietitian who specializes in the FODMAP diet can be extremely beneficial. They can provide personalized guidance, create meal plans, and help you navigate the diet effectively while meeting your nutritional needs.

Remember that the FODMAP diet is highly individual, and what you can tolerate may differ from someone else. It's important to work with a healthcare professional to create a meal plan tailored to your specific needs and monitor your progress and symptoms over time.

FOODS THAT HAVE A CALMING EFFECT ON THE DIGESTIVE SYSTEM AND CAN HELP REDUCE STRESS

Several foods are known for their calming effects on the digestive system and their potential to reduce stress. These foods are typically easy to digest and can promote relaxation. Here are some examples:

• Ginger: Ginger has anti-inflammatory and soothing properties that can help calm the digestive system. It's often used to alleviate nausea and gastrointestinal discomfort.

• Peppermint: Peppermint, in the form of peppermint tea or oil, can relieve indigestion and relax the muscles of the gastrointestinal tract, reducing discomfort.

• Chamomile: Chamomile tea is known for its calming and anti-inflammatory effects on the digestive system. It can help alleviate bloating and soothe an upset stomach.

• Bananas: Bananas are easy to digest and provide a good source of potassium, which can help regulate the digestive system and reduce the impact of stress.

• Oats: Oats are a source of soluble fiber, which can help regulate digestion and reduce inflammation in the gut. They also contain the amino acid tryptophan, which can contribute to a sense of calm.

• Rice: White rice, in particular, is gentle on the digestive system and can be soothing when you have an upset stomach.

• Yogurt: Yogurt, especially plain, unsweetened yogurt with live probiotics, can promote gut health and improve digestion.

• Herbal Teas: Herbal teas like lavender, fennel, and lemon balm can have calming effects on the digestive system and help reduce stress.

• Fennel: Fennel seeds or tea can alleviate digestive discomfort and bloating.

• Papaya: Papaya contains an enzyme called papain, which can aid in digestion and reduce gastrointestinal discomfort.

• Applesauce: Applesauce, especially when made without added sugars, is easy to digest and can help calm the stomach.

• Cooked Vegetables: Steamed or cooked vegetables like carrots, zucchini, and spinach are easier to digest than raw ones and can be gentle on the stomach.

• Miso Soup: Miso is a fermented soybean paste used to make miso soup. It contains probiotics that can promote gut health and digestion.

• Bone Broth: Bone broth is rich in amino acids and minerals that can support digestion and soothe the gut.

It's important to note that while these foods can have a calming effect on the digestive system, individual responses may vary. If you have specific dietary restrictions or medical conditions, it's advisable to consult with a healthcare professional or registered dietitian for personalized guidance on incorporating these foods into your diet. Additionally, the connection between diet and stress is complex, and addressing stress may also require the incorporation of stress-reduction techniques and an overall healthy lifestyle.

THE ROLE OF SUPPLEMENTS AND HERBS, SUCH AS PROBIOTICS, TURMERIC, AND GINGER, IN MANAGING INFLAMMATION.

Supplements and herbs, like probiotics, turmeric, and ginger, have gained attention for their potential role in managing inflammation. It's important to note that while some studies suggest their anti-inflammatory benefits, the efficacy can vary from person to person, and individual results may vary. Here's a discussion of the roles of these supplements and herbs:

1. Probiotics:

• Role: Probiotics are live microorganisms that promote a healthy balance of gut bacteria. They can help modulate the gut microbiome, which plays a significant role in regulating inflammation throughout the body.

• Mechanism: By improving gut health, probiotics can reduce the production of pro-inflammatory cytokines and promote the production of anti-inflammatory compounds.

• Evidence: Several studies suggest that certain strains of probiotics may help reduce inflammation, especially in conditions like irritable bowel syndrome (IBS) and inflammatory bowel disease (IBD).

2. Turmeric (Curcumin):

• Role: Turmeric contains a bioactive compound called curcumin, which is known for its potent anti-inflammatory and antioxidant properties.

• Mechanism: Curcumin inhibits pro-inflammatory pathways in the body, such as the NF-kB pathway. It also scavenges free radicals and reduces oxidative stress.

• Evidence: Numerous studies have demonstrated the anti-inflammatory effects of curcumin. It is often used to alleviate symptoms in conditions like osteoarthritis, rheumatoid arthritis, and inflammatory disorders.

3. Ginger:

• Role: Ginger is a popular spice with anti-inflammatory and analgesic properties. It has been used for centuries to treat various inflammatory conditions.

• Mechanism: Gingerol, the active compound in ginger, exerts its anti-inflammatory effects by inhibiting COX-2, an enzyme responsible for inflammation, and reducing the expression of pro-inflammatory genes.

• Evidence: Research suggests that ginger can help reduce inflammation, especially in conditions like osteoarthritis, muscle pain, and menstrual discomfort.

It's essential to approach the use of supplements and herbs for managing inflammation with caution and consult with a healthcare professional before incorporating them into your routine, especially if you have underlying medical conditions or are taking other medications. Some important considerations include:

• Quality and Dosage: The quality and potency of supplements can vary. Choose reputable brands, and follow recommended dosages.

• Potential Side Effects: Some individuals may experience side effects, particularly with high doses or long-term use. For example, curcumin may interact with certain medications, and ginger may cause gastrointestinal discomfort in high doses.

• Individual Response: The effectiveness of these supplements and herbs can vary from person to person. What works for one individual may not work for another.

• Interaction with Medications: Some supplements and herbs may interact with prescription medications. It's crucial to discuss any potential interactions with your healthcare provider.

In summary, probiotics, turmeric (curcumin), and ginger have shown promise in managing inflammation, and they can be part of a comprehensive approach to reducing inflammation in the body. However, it's important to use them cautiously, in consultation with a healthcare professional, and as part of an overall healthy lifestyle that includes a balanced diet and regular physical activity.

POTENTIAL INTERACTIONS WITH THE FODMAP DIET.

When considering the use of supplements and herbs like probiotics, turmeric, and ginger for managing inflammation in the context of the FODMAP diet, it's essential to be aware of potential interactions and considerations:

1. FODMAP Content:

• Probiotics: Some probiotics may contain FODMAPs or prebiotics, which can exacerbate symptoms in individuals sensitive to these carbohydrates. Check the label for any FODMAP ingredients.

• Turmeric (Curcumin): Turmeric itself is considered low FODMAP in small amounts, but if you're using turmeric supplements or consuming large quantities, it may contain FODMAPs.

• Ginger: Ginger is generally low FODMAP and well-tolerated, but excessive consumption can sometimes lead to gastrointestinal discomfort.

2. Individual Tolerance:

Everyone's tolerance to specific FODMAPs, supplements, and herbs can vary. Some individuals with irritable bowel syndrome (IBS) or other digestive conditions may be more sensitive to certain compounds.

3. Dosage and Form:

The dosage and form in which you take these supplements can influence their FODMAP content and potential for digestive discomfort. For example, high doses of turmeric supplements may contain FODMAPs, while using fresh ginger or ginger capsules may be better tolerated.

4. Interaction with Dietary Changes:

When incorporating these supplements and herbs into your FODMAP diet, be mindful of how they interact with your overall dietary changes. You may need to make adjustments based on your individual response.

5. Consult a Healthcare Professional:

It's advisable to consult with a healthcare professional, such as a registered dietitian or a gastroenterologist, who can provide personalized guidance on incorporating supplements and herbs while following the FODMAP diet. They can help you choose suitable options and tailor your plan to your specific needs.

In summary, while probiotics, turmeric, and ginger can be valuable additions to a diet aimed at managing inflammation, it's important to pay attention to potential FODMAP content and how they interact with the FODMAP diet. Individual tolerance, dosage, and form of these supplements and herbs should be considered, and consulting with a healthcare professional is advisable for those following the FODMAP diet, particularly if they have digestive conditions like IBS.

HOW TO NAVIGATE SOCIAL EVENTS AND DINING OUT WHILE FOLLOWING THE FODMAP DIET AND MANAGING STRESS.

Navigating social events and dining out while following the FODMAP diet and managing stress can be challenging but is entirely manageable with some planning and communication. Here are some tips to help you enjoy these situations without compromising your health and well-being:

1. Plan Ahead:

• Check the Menu: Before attending a social event or dining out, review the menu online if possible. Look for FODMAP-friendly options or ingredients you can tolerate.

• Call Ahead: If you're unsure about the menu or if they can accommodate your dietary needs, call the restaurant or event organizer in advance to discuss your requirements.

• Eat Beforehand: If you're uncertain about the available options, have a small, low-FODMAP meal or snack before going to the event to reduce hunger and temptation.

2. Communicate Clearly:

• Inform Your Host: If you're attending a gathering at someone's home, let your host know about your dietary restrictions. Offer to bring a dish you can enjoy and share with others.

• Speak with the Server: When dining out, communicate your dietary needs to the server. Be polite but clear about your restrictions. They can often assist with modifications or suggestions.

3. Be Mindful of Stress:

• Stress Reduction Techniques: Practice stress reduction techniques, such as deep breathing, mindfulness, or meditation before and during the event to manage any anxiety related to your dietary restrictions.

• Prioritize Social Connection: Focus on the social aspect of the event rather than just the food. Engage in conversations, enjoy the company, and shift your attention away from food-related stress.

4. Choose Wisely:

• Select Low-FODMAP Options: Opt for foods that are naturally low in FODMAPs. Protein-based dishes, salads with safe vegetables, and plain rice or potatoes are often safer choices.

• Ask for Modifications: Don't be afraid to ask for menu modifications, like removing high-FODMAP ingredients or substituting them with low-FODMAP alternatives.

• Avoid Hidden FODMAPs: Be cautious about hidden FODMAP sources like sauces, marinades, and dressings. Request these on the side or inquire about their ingredients.

5. Portable Snacks:

Carry safe, portable low-FODMAP snacks in your bag or pocket, like rice cakes, nuts, or lactose-free cheese, in case suitable food options are limited.

6. Practice Portion Control:

While following the FODMAP diet, even some low-FODMAP foods can cause symptoms if consumed in large quantities. Pay attention to portion sizes.

7. Be Prepared for Questions:

Be ready to explain your dietary choices to curious friends or acquaintances. Educate them about the FODMAP diet if necessary.

8. Enjoy Safe Treats:

If dessert is part of the event, bring your own low-FODMAP dessert to share, so you're not left out of the sweet indulgence.

9. Stay Positive:

Maintain a positive attitude. Remember that managing stress and sticking to your dietary requirements are vital for your well-being, and it's okay to prioritize your health.

10. Reflect and Adapt:

After the event, take time to reflect on your experience. What worked well, and what could be improved for the next time?

Use these insights to refine your approach for future social events.

Remember that it's entirely possible to enjoy social gatherings and dining out while following the FODMAP diet and managing stress. With careful planning, clear communication, and a positive mindset, you can participate in these events without compromising your health or enjoyment.

COMMON CHALLENGES THAT MAY BE ENCOUNTERED WHILE ON THE FODMAP DIET AND MANAGING STRESS AND INFLAMMATION.

Here are some common challenges that may be encountered, along with guidance on how to address them:

1. Difficulty in Identifying FODMAP Sources

Solution: Keep a food diary and work with a registered dietitian who specializes in the FODMAP diet. They can help you pinpoint specific FODMAP sources and offer suitable alternatives.

2. Social Pressure During Events

Solution: Communicate your dietary needs to hosts or restaurant staff ahead of time. Bring a safe dish to share at social gatherings, and focus on the social aspect rather than the food. Educate friends and family about your dietary requirements to ease any social pressure.

3. Managing Stress

Solution: Incorporate stress-reduction techniques into your daily routine, such as mindfulness, meditation, yoga, and deep breathing exercises. Seek support from a therapist or counselor if necessary.

4. Inconsistent Symptom Management

Solution: Symptom management can vary from person to person. It's essential to be patient and consistent with the diet and other lifestyle changes. Consult with a healthcare provider or dietitian to identify specific triggers.

5. Balancing Dietary Restrictions with Nutrient Intake

Solution: Consult with a registered dietitian to create a well-balanced meal plan that meets your nutritional needs while adhering to the FODMAP diet. They can help you choose nutrient-rich, low-FODMAP foods.

PART TWO

Scrambled Eggs with Spinach and Tomatoes

Ingredients:

• 2 large eggs

• 1 cup fresh spinach

• 1 small tomato, diced

• 1 tablespoon garlic-infused olive oil

• Salt and pepper to taste

Instructions:

1. Heat the garlic-infused olive oil in a non-stick skillet over medium heat.

2. Add the diced tomato and cook for 2-3 minutes until it starts to soften. Add the fresh spinach and sauté until wilted.

3. In a bowl, whisk the eggs, then pour them into the skillet.

4. Stir the eggs and cook until they're scrambled to your desired level of doneness.

5. Season with salt and pepper. Serve hot.

Greek Yogurt Parfait

Ingredients:

• 1 cup lactose-free Greek yogurt

• 1/2 cup blueberries

• 1/4 cup strawberries, tops removed and sliced

• 1 tablespoon maple syrup (optional for sweetness)

• 1 tablespoon chopped almonds (optional)

Instructions:

1. In a glass or bowl, layer the lactose-free Greek yogurt, blueberries, and sliced strawberries.

2. Drizzle with maple syrup for sweetness, if desired. Top with chopped almonds.

3. Enjoy your parfait.

Banana and Peanut Butter Smoothie

Ingredients:

• 1 ripe banana (ensure it's not overripe)

• 1 tablespoon peanut butter (with no added high-FODMAP ingredients)

• 1 cup lactose-free or almond milk

• 1/2 cup ice cubes

Instructions:

1. Peel and slice the banana. Place the banana, peanut butter, lactose-free or almond milk, and ice cubes in a blender.

2. Blend until smooth and creamy.

3. Pour into a glass and enjoy your low-FODMAP smoothie.

Quinoa Breakfast Bowl

Ingredients:

• 1/2 cup cooked quinoa

• 1/4 cup sliced strawberries

- 1/4 cup blueberries

- 1 tablespoon chopped pecans

- 1 tablespoon maple syrup (optional for sweetness)

Instructions:

1. Cook quinoa according to package instructions.

2. In a bowl, layer the cooked quinoa, sliced strawberries, and blueberries.

3. Top with chopped pecans and drizzle with maple syrup if desired.

4. Serve and enjoy.

Rice Cake with Almond Butter and Banana

Ingredients:

- 1 rice cake (check the ingredients to ensure it's low-FODMAP)

- 1 tablespoon almond butter

- 1/2 banana, thinly sliced

• A pinch of cinnamon (optional)

Instructions:

1. Spread almond butter evenly on the rice cake. Top with thinly sliced banana.

2. Sprinkle a pinch of cinnamon for extra flavor if desired.

3. Enjoy your simple and quick low-FODMAP breakfast.

Spinach and Bacon Omelette

Ingredients:

• 2 large eggs

• 1 cup fresh spinach

• 2 strips of cooked bacon, crumbled

• 1 tablespoon lactose-free milk

• Salt and pepper to taste

Instructions:

1. In a bowl, whisk the eggs and lactose-free milk.

2. Heat a non-stick skillet over medium heat and add a small amount of olive oil or non-dairy margarine.

3. Add fresh spinach to the skillet and sauté until wilted. Pour the egg mixture over the spinach.

4. Sprinkle the crumbled bacon on top. Cook until the eggs are set and slightly golden on the bottom.

5. Fold the omelette in half and serve.

Chia Seed Pudding with Berries

Ingredients:

• 2 tablespoons chia seeds

• 1 cup lactose-free or almond milk

• 1/2 cup mixed low-FODMAP berries (e.g., blueberries, strawberries)

• 1/2 tablespoon maple syrup (optional for sweetness)

Instructions:

1. In a jar or bowl, mix chia seeds and milk. Stir well and refrigerate for at least 2 hours or overnight to let it thicken.

2. In the morning, top with mixed berries. Drizzle with maple syrup for added sweetness if desired.

3. Enjoy your chia seed pudding.

Low-FODMAP Pancakes

Ingredients:

• 1 cup gluten-free flour mix (ensure it's FODMAP-friendly)

• 1 teaspoon baking powder

• 1 large egg

• 1 cup lactose-free milk

• 1 tablespoon vegetable oil

• 1 tablespoon maple syrup (optional)

• Cooking spray (for the skillet)

Instructions:

1. In a bowl, combine the gluten-free flour and baking powder.

2. In a separate bowl, whisk the egg, lactose-free milk, vegetable oil, and maple syrup. Pour the wet ingredients into the dry ingredients and mix until well combined.

3. Heat a non-stick skillet over medium heat and lightly grease it with cooking spray. Pour pancake batter onto the skillet, using 1/4 cup for each pancake.

4. Cook until bubbles form on the surface, then flip and cook until golden brown.

5. Serve with maple syrup or other low-FODMAP toppings.

Smoked Salmon and Dill Rice Cakes

Ingredients:

• 2 rice cakes (check ingredients to ensure they're low-FODMAP)

• 2 ounces smoked salmon

• 1 tablespoon lactose-free cream cheese

• Fresh dill, for garnish

Instructions:

1. Spread lactose-free cream cheese evenly on each rice cake.

2. Top with smoked salmon and garnish with fresh dill.

3. Enjoy your simple and savory breakfast.

Quinoa and Zucchini Fritters

Ingredients:

• 1 cup cooked quinoa

• 1 small zucchini, grated and excess moisture squeezed out

• 1 egg

• 1/4 cup gluten-free breadcrumbs (check ingredients)

• 1 tablespoon chopped chives

• Salt and pepper to taste

• Olive oil for cooking

Instructions:

1. In a bowl, combine cooked quinoa, grated zucchini, egg, gluten-free breadcrumbs, and chopped chives.

2. Season with salt and pepper. Form the mixture into small fritters.

3. Heat olive oil in a skillet over medium heat and cook the fritters until golden brown on both sides.

4. Serve with a side of lactose-free yogurt or a low-FODMAP sauce.

Peanut Butter Banana Rice Cakes

Ingredients:

• 2 rice cakes (check the ingredients to ensure they're low-FODMAP)

• 2 tablespoons peanut butter (with no added high-FODMAP ingredients)

• 1 small ripe banana, sliced

• A pinch of cinnamon (optional)

Instructions:

1. Spread peanut butter evenly on each rice cake. Top with banana slices.

2. Sprinkle a pinch of cinnamon for extra flavor if desired.

3. Enjoy your quick and satisfying breakfast.

Lactose-Free Yogurt and Berry Parfait

Ingredients:

• 1 cup lactose-free yogurt

• 1/2 cup mixed low-FODMAP berries (e.g., blueberries, strawberries)

• 2 tablespoons gluten-free granola (check ingredients)

• 1 tablespoon maple syrup (optional for sweetness)

Instructions:

1. In a glass or bowl, layer the lactose-free yogurt, mixed berries, and gluten-free granola.

2. Drizzle with maple syrup for added sweetness if desired.

3. Serve and enjoy your yogurt parfait.

Sweet Potato and Zucchini Hash

Ingredients:

- 1 small sweet potato, peeled and diced

- 1 small zucchini, diced

- 2 eggs

- 1 tablespoon garlic-infused olive oil

- Salt and pepper to taste

- Fresh chives for garnish

Instructions:

1. Heat the garlic-infused olive oil in a skillet over medium heat.

2. Add the diced sweet potato and cook for 5-7 minutes, or until it begins to soften. Add the diced zucchini and cook for an additional 5 minutes.

3. Create two wells in the hash mixture and crack an egg into each well. Cover the skillet and cook until the eggs are cooked to your desired level.

4. Season with salt and pepper, and garnish with fresh chives.

5. Serve hot.

Oatmeal with Maple and Pecans

Ingredients:

• 1/2 cup rolled oats (ensure they're gluten-free and low-FODMAP)

• 1 cup lactose-free milk

• 1 tablespoon maple syrup

• 1 tablespoon chopped pecans

• A pinch of cinnamon (optional)

Instructions:

1. In a saucepan, combine the rolled oats and lactose-free milk.

2. Cook over medium heat, stirring, until the oats are creamy and fully cooked. Stir in maple syrup and remove from heat.

3. Top with chopped pecans and a pinch of cinnamon if desired.

4. Enjoy your warm and comforting oatmeal.

Low-FODMAP Smoothie Bowl

Ingredients:

• 1 cup lactose-free yogurt

• 1/2 cup mixed low-FODMAP berries (e.g., blueberries, strawberries)

• 1 small banana (ensure it's not overripe)

• 2 tablespoons gluten-free granola (check ingredients)

• 1 tablespoon chia seeds (optional)

Instructions:

1. In a bowl, layer lactose-free yogurt, mixed berries, and sliced banana.

2. Sprinkle gluten-free granola and chia seeds on top. Customize with additional low-FODMAP toppings of your choice.

3. Enjoy your nutritious and visually appealing smoothie bowl.

Frittata with Spinach and Feta

Ingredients:

• 4 large eggs

• 1 cup fresh spinach

• 1/4 cup crumbled lactose-free feta cheese

• 1 tablespoon garlic-infused olive oil

• Salt and pepper to taste

Instructions:

1. Preheat the oven to 350°F (175°C).

2. In an oven-safe skillet, heat the garlic-infused olive oil over medium heat. Add fresh spinach and cook until wilted.

3. In a bowl, whisk the eggs, salt, and pepper. Pour the egg mixture into the skillet over the spinach.

4. Sprinkle crumbled lactose-free feta cheese on top.

5. Transfer the skillet to the oven and bake for about 15-20 minutes, until the frittata is set and lightly golden.

6. Slice and serve.

Polenta with Sautéed Spinach and Tomatoes

Ingredients:

• 1/2 cup instant polenta

• 2 cups water

• 1 cup fresh spinach

• 1 small tomato, diced

• 1 tablespoon garlic-infused olive oil

• Salt and pepper to taste

Instructions:

1. In a saucepan, bring 2 cups of water to a boil. Gradually whisk in the instant polenta, reduce heat, and cook according to package instructions.

2. In a skillet, heat the garlic-infused olive oil over medium heat.

3. Add diced tomato and sauté for 2-3 minutes. Add fresh spinach and cook until wilted.

4. Season with salt and pepper.

5. Serve the sautéed spinach and tomatoes over a bed of cooked polenta.

Low-FODMAP Breakfast Burrito

Ingredients:

- 2 corn tortillas (check ingredients)

- 2 scrambled eggs

- 2 slices of cooked bacon, crumbled

- 1/4 cup diced bell peppers

- 1/4 cup diced tomatoes

- 2 tablespoons salsa (ensure it's low-FODMAP)

Instructions:

1. Warm the corn tortillas in a dry skillet for a few seconds on each side.

2. Fill each tortilla with scrambled eggs, crumbled bacon, diced bell peppers, diced tomatoes, and a dollop of salsa.

3. Roll up the tortillas into burritos.

4. Serve and enjoy.

Low-FODMAP Avocado Toast

Ingredients:

• 2 slices of gluten-free bread (check ingredients)

• 1/2 ripe avocado, mashed

• A pinch of salt

• Chopped chives (green tops only) for garnish

Instructions:

1. Toast the gluten-free bread. Spread the mashed avocado evenly on the toast.

2. Sprinkle with a pinch of salt and garnish with chopped chives (green tops).

3. Enjoy your simple and nutritious avocado toast.

Ingredients:

• 1 cup mashed potatoes (prepared without high-FODMAP ingredients)

• 2 slices of cooked bacon, crumbled

• 1 fried or poached egg

• Fresh chives (green tops only) for garnish

Instructions:

1. Reheat or prepare mashed potatoes. Place the mashed potatoes in a bowl.

2. Top with crumbled bacon. Add a fried or poached egg on top.

3. Garnish with fresh chives (green tops). Serve your hearty breakfast bowl.

Quinoa Breakfast Bowl with Berries and Almonds

Ingredients:

- 1/2 cup cooked quinoa

- 1/4 cup mixed low-FODMAP berries (e.g., blueberries, raspberries)

- 1 tablespoon chopped almonds

- 1 tablespoon maple syrup (optional)

Instructions:

1. Cook quinoa according to package instructions.

2. In a bowl, layer the cooked quinoa, mixed berries, and chopped almonds. Drizzle with maple syrup for added sweetness, if desired.

3. Enjoy your protein-rich and satisfying breakfast bowl.

Rice Cake with Lactose-Free Cream Cheese and Smoked Salmon

Ingredients:

- 1 rice cake (check ingredients to ensure it's low-FODMAP)

- 2 tablespoons lactose-free cream cheese

- 2 slices of smoked salmon

- Fresh dill for garnish

Instructions:

1. Spread lactose-free cream cheese evenly on the rice cake.

2. Top with smoked salmon. Garnish with fresh dill.

3. Enjoy your elegant and flavorful breakfast option.

Blueberry Pancakes (Low-FODMAP)

Ingredients:

- 1 cup gluten-free flour mix (ensure it's low-FODMAP)

- 1 teaspoon baking powder

- 1 large egg

- 1 cup lactose-free milk

- 1 cup fresh blueberries

- Cooking spray (for the skillet)

Instructions:

1. In a bowl, combine gluten-free flour and baking powder.

2. In a separate bowl, whisk the egg and lactose-free milk. Pour the wet ingredients into the dry ingredients and mix until well combined.

3. Gently fold in the fresh blueberries.

4. Heat a non-stick skillet over medium heat and lightly grease it with cooking spray. Pour pancake batter onto the skillet, using 1/4 cup for each pancake.

5. Cook until bubbles form on the surface, then flip and cook until golden brown.

6. Serve with maple syrup or other low-FODMAP toppings.

Low-FODMAP Grilled Chicken and Quinoa Salad

Ingredients:

• 1 cup cooked quinoa

• 4 oz grilled chicken breast, sliced

• 1 cup mixed salad greens (e.g., spinach, arugula)

• 1/4 cup cherry tomatoes

• 1/4 cup cucumber, sliced

• 1 tablespoon FODMAP-friendly vinaigrette dressing

Instructions:

1. In a large bowl, combine cooked quinoa and mixed salad greens.

2. Add grilled chicken, cherry tomatoes, and cucumber. Drizzle with the FODMAP-friendly vinaigrette dressing.

3. Toss gently to combine, and enjoy your nutritious and satisfying salad.

Ingredients:

• 1 cup cooked quinoa

• 1 can (5 oz) canned tuna, drained

• 1/4 cup red bell pepper, diced

• 1/4 cup carrots, grated

• 1/4 cup fresh spinach

• 2 tablespoons olive oil

• 1 tablespoon rice wine vinegar

• Salt and pepper to taste

Instructions:

1. In a bowl, combine cooked quinoa, canned tuna, diced red bell pepper, grated carrots, and fresh spinach.

2. In a separate small bowl, whisk together olive oil, rice wine vinegar, salt, and pepper to create a dressing.

3. Drizzle the dressing over the salad and toss to combine.

4. Enjoy your protein-packed quinoa and tuna salad.

Low-FODMAP Baked Salmon with Lemon and Asparagus

Ingredients:

• 1 salmon fillet

• 8-10 asparagus spears

• 1 lemon, thinly sliced

• 1 tablespoon garlic-infused olive oil

• Salt and pepper to taste

Instructions:

1. Preheat the oven to 375°F (190°C).

2. Place the salmon fillet on a baking sheet lined with aluminum foil. Arrange asparagus spears around the salmon.

3. Drizzle garlic-infused olive oil over the salmon and asparagus. Season with salt and pepper.

4. Place lemon slices on top of the salmon. Bake in the preheated oven for 15-20 minutes or until the salmon is cooked through.

5. Serve hot with a side of low-FODMAP vegetables or rice.

Low-FODMAP Turkey and Lettuce Wraps

Ingredients:

• 1/2 lb ground turkey

• 1/4 cup diced red bell pepper

• 1/4 cup diced cucumber

• 1/4 cup green leaf lettuce leaves

• 1 tablespoon garlic-infused olive oil

• 1 tablespoon low-FODMAP hoisin sauce

• Salt and pepper to taste

Instructions:

1. In a skillet, heat garlic-infused olive oil over medium heat.

2. Add ground turkey and cook until browned and cooked through. Stir in diced red bell pepper and cucumber and sauté for a few minutes.

3. Season with salt and pepper and mix in the low-FODMAP hoisin sauce. Spoon the turkey mixture into lettuce leaves to create wraps.

4. Serve your tasty and low-FODMAP lettuce wraps.

Low-FODMAP Tomato and Basil Quinoa Bowl

Ingredients:

• 1 cup cooked quinoa

• 1/4 cup diced tomatoes

• 1/4 cup fresh basil leaves

• 1 tablespoon garlic-infused olive oil

• 1 tablespoon balsamic vinegar

• Salt and pepper to taste

Instructions:

1. In a bowl, combine cooked quinoa, diced tomatoes, and fresh basil leaves.

2. In a separate small bowl, whisk together garlic-infused olive oil, balsamic vinegar, salt, and pepper to create a dressing.

3. Drizzle the dressing over the quinoa bowl and toss to combine.

4. Enjoy your light and refreshing tomato and basil quinoa bowl.

Low-FODMAP Turkey and Spinach Stuffed Peppers

Ingredients:

• 2 bell peppers (choose red, yellow, or green)

• 1/2 lb ground turkey

• 1 cup fresh spinach

• 1/4 cup diced tomatoes

• 1/4 cup shredded lactose-free cheddar cheese

• 1 tablespoon garlic-infused olive oil

• Salt and pepper to taste

Instructions:

1. Preheat the oven to 375°F (190°C).

2. Cut the tops off the bell peppers and remove the seeds and membranes.

3. In a skillet, heat garlic-infused olive oil over medium heat. Add ground turkey and cook until browned and cooked through.

4. Stir in fresh spinach and diced tomatoes and sauté for a few minutes. Season with salt and pepper.

5. Spoon the turkey and spinach mixture into the bell peppers. Top with shredded lactose-free cheddar cheese.

6. Place the stuffed peppers in a baking dish and bake for 25-30 minutes or until the peppers are tender.

7. Serve your delicious stuffed peppers.

Low-FODMAP Quinoa and Mixed Vegetable Stir-Fry

Ingredients:

- 1 cup cooked quinoa

- 1/2 cup mixed low-FODMAP vegetables (e.g., zucchini, bell peppers, carrots)

- 4 oz firm tofu, cubed

- 1 tablespoon garlic-infused olive oil

- 2 tablespoons low-sodium soy sauce (check for FODMAP-friendly options)

- 1 tablespoon sesame seeds

Instructions:

1. In a skillet, heat garlic-infused olive oil over medium heat.

2. Add mixed vegetables and tofu cubes and stir-fry until the vegetables are tender and the tofu is lightly browned.

3. Add cooked quinoa to the skillet and drizzle with low-sodium soy sauce.

4. Stir-fry until everything is well combined.

5. Sprinkle sesame seeds on top and serve your flavorful stir-fry.

Low-FODMAP Tuna and Avocado Salad

Ingredients:

• 1 can (5 oz) canned tuna, drained

• 1 small avocado, diced

• 1/4 cup diced red bell pepper

• 1/4 cup diced cucumber

• 1 tablespoon garlic-infused olive oil

• 1 tablespoon lemon juice

• Salt and pepper to taste

Instructions:

1. In a bowl, combine canned tuna, diced avocado, diced red bell pepper, and diced cucumber.

2. In a separate small bowl, whisk together garlic-infused olive oil, lemon juice, salt, and pepper to create a dressing.

3. Drizzle the dressing over the salad and toss to combine.

4. Enjoy your creamy and nutritious tuna and avocado salad.

Low-FODMAP Egg Salad Lettuce Wraps

Ingredients:

• 4 hard-boiled eggs, chopped

• 1/4 cup diced red bell pepper

• 1/4 cup diced carrots

• 4 large lettuce leaves (e.g., iceberg or butter lettuce)

• 2 tablespoons mayonnaise (check for FODMAP-friendly options)

• 1 tablespoon Dijon mustard (ensure it's low-FODMAP)

• Salt and pepper to taste

Instructions:

1. In a bowl, combine chopped hard-boiled eggs, diced red bell pepper, and diced carrots.

2. In a separate small bowl, mix mayonnaise and Dijon mustard to create the dressing.

3. Add the dressing to the egg salad and toss to coat. Spoon the egg salad into large lettuce leaves to create wraps.

4. Serve your tasty and low-FODMAP lettuce wraps.

Low-FODMAP Spaghetti with Basil Pesto

Ingredients:

• 2 oz gluten-free and low-FODMAP spaghetti (check ingredients)

• 1 cup fresh basil leaves

• 1/4 cup pine nuts

• 1/4 cup grated lactose-free Parmesan cheese

• 1/4 cup garlic-infused olive oil

• Salt and pepper to taste

Instructions:

1. Cook the gluten-free spaghetti according to package instructions.

2. In a blender or food processor, combine fresh basil leaves, pine nuts, grated lactose-free Parmesan cheese, and garlic-infused olive oil.

3. Blend until you have a smooth basil pesto sauce. Toss the cooked spaghetti with the basil pesto sauce.

4. Season with salt and pepper.

5. Serve your delightful low-FODMAP spaghetti with basil pesto.

Low-FODMAP Chicken and Rice Soup

Ingredients:

• 4 cups low-FODMAP chicken broth

• 1 cup cooked white rice (ensure it's low-FODMAP)

• 1 cup cooked chicken breast, shredded

• 1/2 cup diced carrots

- 1/2 cup diced zucchini

- Salt and pepper to taste

- Fresh chives (green parts only) for garnish

Instructions:

1. In a large pot, combine low-FODMAP chicken broth, cooked white rice, cooked chicken breast, diced carrots, and diced zucchini.

2. Bring the soup to a simmer and cook for about 10-15 minutes until the vegetables are tender.

3. Season with salt and pepper. Garnish with fresh chives (green parts only).

4. Enjoy your comforting and warming chicken and rice soup.

Low-FODMAP Shrimp and Vegetable Stir-Fry

Ingredients:

- 8 oz shrimp, peeled and deveined

• 1/2 cup mixed low-FODMAP vegetables (e.g., bell peppers, bok choy, carrots)

• 1 cup cooked quinoa (ensure it's low-FODMAP)

• 2 tablespoons garlic-infused olive oil

• 2 tablespoons low-sodium soy sauce (check for FODMAP-friendly options)

• 1 tablespoon sesame seeds

Instructions:

1. In a skillet, heat garlic-infused olive oil over medium heat.

2. Add shrimp and stir-fry until pink and cooked through. Add mixed vegetables and stir-fry until they are tender.

3. Stir in cooked quinoa and drizzle with low-sodium soy sauce. Toss to combine.

4. Sprinkle sesame seeds on top and serve your flavorful stir-fry.

Low-FODMAP Caprese Salad

Ingredients:

• 2 ripe tomatoes, sliced

• 4 oz lactose-free mozzarella cheese, sliced

• Fresh basil leaves

• 1 tablespoon garlic-infused olive oil

• Balsamic vinegar (ensure it's low-FODMAP)

• Salt and pepper to taste

Instructions:

1. Arrange tomato slices and lactose-free mozzarella cheese on a serving platter.

2. Tuck fresh basil leaves between the tomato and cheese slices. Drizzle with garlic-infused olive oil and balsamic vinegar.

3. Season with salt and pepper.

4. Enjoy your classic and refreshing Caprese salad.

Low-FODMAP Tofu and Veggie Rice Bowl

Ingredients:

• 8 oz firm tofu, cubed

• 1/2 cup mixed low-FODMAP vegetables (e.g., zucchini, bell peppers, carrots)

• 1 cup cooked rice (ensure it's low-FODMAP)

• 2 tablespoons garlic-infused olive oil

• 2 tablespoons low-sodium soy sauce (check for FODMAP-friendly options)

• 1 tablespoon sesame seeds

Instructions:

1. In a skillet, heat garlic-infused olive oil over medium heat.

2. Add cubed tofu and cook until lightly browned. Add mixed vegetables and stir-fry until they are tender.

3. Stir in cooked rice and drizzle with low-sodium soy sauce. Toss to combine.

4. Sprinkle sesame seeds on top and serve your flavorful tofu and veggie rice bowl.

Low-FODMAP Salmon and Cucumber Salad

Ingredients:

• 2 salmon fillets

• 1 cucumber, thinly sliced

• 1 tablespoon garlic-infused olive oil

• 1 tablespoon lemon juice

• Dill for garnish

• Salt and pepper to taste

Instructions:

1. Preheat the oven to 375°F (190°C).

2. Season salmon fillets with salt and pepper. Place the salmon on a baking sheet lined with aluminum foil.

3. Bake for about 15-20 minutes or until the salmon is cooked through.

4. While the salmon is baking, combine sliced cucumber, garlic-infused olive oil, lemon juice, and dill in a bowl.

5. When the salmon is done, let it cool slightly and then flake it into the cucumber salad.

6. Toss to combine and serve your delicious salmon and cucumber salad.

Low-FODMAP Turkey and Cranberry Lettuce Wraps

Ingredients:

• 1/2 lb ground turkey

• 1/4 cup cranberry sauce (check for FODMAP-friendly options)

• 1/4 cup diced red bell pepper

• 4 large lettuce leaves (e.g., iceberg or butter lettuce)

• Salt and pepper to taste

Instructions:

1. In a skillet, cook ground turkey until browned and cooked through.

2. Add diced red bell pepper and sauté until tender. Season with salt and pepper.

3. In a bowl, combine cooked turkey, cranberry sauce, and diced red bell pepper. Spoon the turkey mixture into lettuce leaves to create wraps.

4. Serve your delicious and sweet-savory lettuce wraps.

Low-FODMAP Greek Salad with Grilled Chicken

Ingredients:

• 4 oz grilled chicken breast, sliced

• 1 cup mixed salad greens (e.g., romaine, spinach)

• 1/4 cup diced cucumber

• 1/4 cup diced red bell pepper

• 1/4 cup Kalamata olives

• 1/4 cup crumbled lactose-free feta cheese

- 1 tablespoon garlic-infused olive oil

- Salt and pepper to taste

Instructions:

1. In a large bowl, combine mixed salad greens, diced cucumber, diced red bell pepper, Kalamata olives, and crumbled lactose-free feta cheese.

2. Add grilled chicken slices. Drizzle with garlic-infused olive oil.

3. Season with salt and pepper. Toss gently to combine and enjoy your Mediterranean-inspired salad.

Low-FODMAP Sushi Bowl

Ingredients:

- 1 cup cooked sushi rice (ensure it's low-FODMAP)

- 4 oz cooked and sliced seafood (e.g., shrimp, crab, or fish)

- 1/4 cup sliced cucumber

- 1/4 cup sliced carrots

• 2 tablespoons low-sodium soy sauce (check for FODMAP-friendly options)

• Wasabi and pickled ginger (optional)

Instructions:

1. In a bowl, layer cooked sushi rice, sliced seafood, sliced cucumber, and sliced carrots.

2. Drizzle with low-sodium soy sauce. Add a small amount of wasabi and pickled ginger if desired.

3. Enjoy the flavors of sushi in a convenient bowl.

Low-FODMAP Tuna and Spinach Salad

Ingredients:

• 1 can (5 oz) canned tuna, drained

• 1 cup fresh spinach

• 1/4 cup diced tomatoes

• 1/4 cup diced cucumber

• 1 tablespoon garlic-infused olive oil

- 1 tablespoon balsamic vinegar (ensure it's low-FODMAP)

- Salt and pepper to taste

Instructions:

1. In a bowl, combine canned tuna, fresh spinach, diced tomatoes, and diced cucumber.

2. In a separate small bowl, whisk together garlic-infused olive oil, balsamic vinegar, salt, and pepper to create a dressing.

3. Drizzle the dressing over the salad and toss to combine.

4. Enjoy your protein-packed and flavorful tuna and spinach salad.

Low-FODMAP Beef and Broccoli Stir-Fry

Ingredients:

- 8 oz beef strips

- 1/2 cup broccoli florets

- 1 cup cooked quinoa (ensure it's low-FODMAP)

- 2 tablespoons garlic-infused olive oil

• 2 tablespoons low-sodium soy sauce (check for FODMAP-friendly options)

• Sesame seeds for garnish

• Salt and pepper to taste

Instructions:

1. In a skillet, heat garlic-infused olive oil over medium heat.

2. Add beef strips and cook until browned. Add broccoli florets and stir-fry until tender.

3. Stir in cooked quinoa and drizzle with low-sodium soy sauce. Toss to combine.

4. Garnish with sesame seeds and serve your savory beef and broccoli stir-fry.

Low-FODMAP Chicken and Zucchini Noodles

Ingredients:

• 1 boneless, skinless chicken breast

• 2 zucchinis, spiralized into noodles

- 1 tablespoon garlic-infused olive oil

- 1/4 cup diced tomatoes

- 1/4 cup diced red bell pepper

- Salt and pepper to taste

- Fresh basil for garnish

Instructions:

1. In a skillet, heat garlic-infused olive oil over medium heat.

2. Cook the chicken breast until it's no longer pink in the center. Remove the cooked chicken from the skillet and set it aside.

3. In the same skillet, add zucchini noodles, diced tomatoes, and diced red bell pepper. Sauté until the noodles are tender.

4. Slice the cooked chicken and add it back to the skillet. Season with salt and pepper.

5. Garnish with fresh basil and serve your flavorful chicken and zucchini noodle dish.

Low-FODMAP Tofu and Vegetable Rice Paper Rolls

Ingredients:

• Rice paper wrappers (ensure they're low-FODMAP)

• 4 oz firm tofu, cut into thin strips

• 1/4 cup mixed low-FODMAP vegetables (e.g., cucumber, bell pepper, carrots)

• Fresh basil leaves

• Dipping sauce (prepare with low-FODMAP ingredients)

Instructions:

1. Dip a rice paper wrapper into warm water to soften it.

2. Place the softened wrapper on a flat surface. Arrange strips of tofu, mixed vegetables, and fresh basil leaves in the center.

3. Fold in the sides of the wrapper and roll it up tightly. Repeat with the remaining wrappers and fillings.

4. Serve with your prepared low-FODMAP dipping sauce.

Low-FODMAP Shrimp and Avocado Salad

Ingredients:

• 8 oz cooked and peeled shrimp

• 1 small avocado, diced

• 1/4 cup diced cucumber

• 1/4 cup diced red bell pepper

• 1 tablespoon garlic-infused olive oil

• 1 tablespoon lemon juice

• Salt and pepper to taste

Instructions:

1. In a bowl, combine cooked shrimp, diced avocado, diced cucumber, and diced red bell pepper.

2. In a separate small bowl, whisk together garlic-infused olive oil, lemon juice, salt, and pepper to create a dressing.

3. Drizzle the dressing over the salad and toss to combine.

4. Enjoy your protein-packed and creamy shrimp and avocado salad.

Low-FODMAP Spinach and Bacon Salad

Ingredients:

• 2 cups fresh spinach

• 4 strips of cooked bacon, crumbled

• 1/4 cup diced tomatoes

• 1/4 cup diced cucumber

• 1 tablespoon garlic-infused olive oil

• 1 tablespoon balsamic vinegar (ensure it's low-FODMAP)

• Salt and pepper to taste

Instructions:

1. In a large bowl, combine fresh spinach, crumbled bacon, diced tomatoes, and diced cucumber.

2. In a separate small bowl, whisk together garlic-infused olive oil, balsamic vinegar, salt, and pepper to create a dressing.

3. Drizzle the dressing over the salad and toss to combine.

4. Enjoy your hearty and savory spinach and bacon salad.

Low-FODMAP Shrimp and Quinoa Stir-Fry

Ingredients:

• 8 oz cooked shrimp

• 1 cup cooked quinoa (ensure it's low-FODMAP)

• 1/4 cup diced red bell pepper

• 1/4 cup sliced scallions (green parts only)

• 2 tablespoons garlic-infused olive oil

• 2 tablespoons low-sodium soy sauce (check for FODMAP-friendly options)

• Salt and pepper to taste

Instructions:

1. In a skillet, heat garlic-infused olive oil over medium heat.

2. Add cooked shrimp and sauté until heated through. Stir in cooked quinoa, diced red bell pepper, and sliced scallions.

3. Drizzle with low-sodium soy sauce. Toss to combine. Season with salt and pepper.

4. Serve your flavorful shrimp and quinoa stir-fry.

Low-FODMAP BBQ Chicken and Corn on the Cob

Ingredients:

• 4 bone-in, skin-on chicken thighs

• 4 ears of corn, husked

• 1/2 cup low-FODMAP BBQ sauce

• 2 tablespoons garlic-infused olive oil

• Salt and pepper to taste

Instructions:

1. Preheat the grill to medium-high heat. Season chicken thighs with salt and pepper.

2. Brush with garlic-infused olive oil and grill for about 6-8 minutes per side, or until they are cooked through.

3. In the last 10 minutes of grilling, place the ears of corn on the grill and rotate occasionally until they are slightly charred.

4. Brush the grilled chicken with low-FODMAP BBQ sauce and serve with the grilled corn.

Low-FODMAP Thai Green Curry with Shrimp

Ingredients:

• 8 oz large shrimp, peeled and deveined

• 1 cup mixed low-FODMAP vegetables (e.g., bell peppers, zucchini, carrots)

• 1 can (14 oz) low-fat coconut milk

• 2 tablespoons green curry paste (check for FODMAP-friendly options)

• 2 tablespoons garlic-infused olive oil

• Salt and pepper to taste

• Fresh cilantro for garnish

• Cooked rice (ensure it's low-FODMAP)

Instructions:

1. In a large skillet, heat garlic-infused olive oil over medium heat.

2. Add shrimp and cook until they turn pink. Add mixed vegetables and stir-fry until they are tender.

3. Stir in green curry paste and sauté for a minute. Pour in low-fat coconut milk and let the mixture simmer for 10-15 minutes.

4. Season with salt and pepper. Serve the Thai green curry with shrimp over cooked rice and garnish with fresh cilantro.

Low-FODMAP Beef and Zucchini Stir-Fry

Ingredients:

• 1/2 lb lean beef, thinly sliced

• 2 medium zucchinis, sliced into rounds

• 2 tablespoons garlic-infused olive oil

• 2 tablespoons low-sodium soy sauce (check for FODMAP-friendly options)

- 1 tablespoon fresh ginger, minced

- Salt and pepper to taste

Instructions:

1. In a wok or skillet, heat garlic-infused olive oil over high heat.

2. Add thinly sliced beef and cook until browned. Add zucchini rounds and stir-fry until they are tender.

3. Stir in fresh ginger and sauté for a minute. Drizzle with low-sodium soy sauce and season with salt and pepper.

4. Toss to combine and serve your flavorful beef and zucchini stir-fry with rice or rice noodles.

Low-FODMAP Lemon and Dill Grilled Swordfish

Ingredients:

- 4 swordfish steaks

- Zest and juice of 1 lemon

- 2 tablespoons garlic-infused olive oil

- 2 tablespoons fresh dill, chopped

• Salt and pepper to taste

Instructions:

1. In a bowl, combine lemon zest, lemon juice, garlic-infused olive oil, fresh dill, salt, and pepper.

2. Brush the swordfish steaks with this mixture and let them marinate for at least 30 minutes.

3. Preheat the grill to medium-high heat. Grill the swordfish for about 3-4 minutes per side, or until they are cooked through and have grill marks.

4. Serve your lemon and dill grilled swordfish with a side of quinoa or a green salad.

Low-FODMAP Stuffed Bell Peppers with Turkey

Ingredients:

• 4 large bell peppers

• 1/2 lb ground turkey

• 1 cup cooked rice (ensure it's low-FODMAP)

- 1/4 cup diced tomatoes

- 1/4 cup diced zucchini

- 1/4 cup diced carrots

- 2 tablespoons garlic-infused olive oil

- Salt and pepper to taste

Instructions:

1. Preheat the oven to 350°F (175°C). Cut the tops off the bell peppers and remove the seeds.

2. In a skillet, heat garlic-infused olive oil over medium heat. Add ground turkey and cook until browned.

3. Stir in cooked rice, diced tomatoes, diced zucchini, and diced carrots. Season with salt and pepper.

4. Stuff the bell peppers with the turkey and rice mixture. Place the stuffed peppers in a baking dish and bake for 30-35 minutes.

5. Serve your delicious stuffed bell peppers as a main dish or side.

Low-FODMAP Grilled Shrimp and Pineapple Skewers

Ingredients:

• 8 oz large shrimp, peeled and deveined

• 2 cups pineapple chunks

• 2 tablespoons garlic-infused olive oil

• 1 tablespoon fresh cilantro, chopped

• Salt and pepper to taste

Instructions:

1. Preheat the grill to medium-high heat.

2. Thread the shrimp and pineapple chunks onto skewers, alternating between them.

3. In a bowl, combine garlic-infused olive oil, fresh cilantro, salt, and pepper. Brush the skewers with the cilantro mixture.

4. Grill the skewers for about 2-3 minutes on each side, or until the shrimp are pink and cooked through.

5. Serve your grilled shrimp and pineapple skewers with rice or a side salad.

Low-FODMAP Caprese Quinoa Salad

Ingredients:

• 2 cups cooked quinoa (ensure it's low-FODMAP)

• 1 cup cherry tomatoes, halved

• 1 cup fresh mozzarella cheese, cubed

• 1/4 cup fresh basil leaves

• 2 tablespoons garlic-infused olive oil

• Balsamic vinegar (check for FODMAP-friendly options)

• Salt and pepper to taste

Instructions:

1. In a large bowl, combine cooked quinoa, cherry tomatoes, fresh mozzarella cheese, and fresh basil leaves.

2. Drizzle with garlic-infused olive oil and balsamic vinegar. Season with salt and pepper.

3. Toss to combine and serve your refreshing Caprese quinoa salad.

Low-FODMAP Lemon Herb Roasted Chicken

Ingredients:

• 4 bone-in, skin-on chicken thighs

• Zest and juice of 1 lemon

• 2 tablespoons garlic-infused olive oil

• 2 tablespoons fresh rosemary, chopped

• Salt and pepper to taste

Instructions:

1. Preheat the oven to 375°F (190°C).

2. In a bowl, combine lemon zest, lemon juice, garlic-infused olive oil, fresh rosemary, salt, and pepper.

3. Place the chicken thighs in a baking dish and brush them with the lemon and herb mixture.

4. Roast in the oven for 35-40 minutes or until the chicken is golden and fully cooked.

5. Serve with a low-FODMAP side, such as quinoa or sautéed spinach.

Low-FODMAP Teriyaki Tofu and Vegetable Stir-Fry

Ingredients:

- 8 oz extra-firm tofu, cubed

- 2 cups mixed low-FODMAP vegetables (e.g., bell peppers, snap peas, carrots)

- 2 tablespoons garlic-infused olive oil

- 2 tablespoons low-sodium soy sauce (check for FODMAP-friendly options)

- 1 tablespoon fresh ginger, minced

- Salt and pepper to taste

Instructions:

1. In a wok or large skillet, heat garlic-infused olive oil over high heat.

2. Add cubed tofu and stir-fry until it's lightly browned. Add mixed vegetables and continue stir-frying until they are tender.

3. Stir in fresh ginger and cook for a minute. Drizzle with low-sodium soy sauce and season with salt and pepper.

4. Toss to combine and serve the teriyaki tofu and vegetable stir-fry with rice or rice noodles.

Low-FODMAP Tomato and Basil Grilled Chicken

Ingredients:

• 4 boneless, skinless chicken breasts

• 2 tablespoons garlic-infused olive oil

• 1 cup cherry tomatoes, halved

• 1/4 cup fresh basil leaves

• Salt and pepper to taste

Instructions:

1. Preheat the grill to medium-high heat. Season chicken breasts with salt and pepper.

2. Brush with garlic-infused olive oil. Grill the chicken for 6-8 minutes per side or until they are cooked through.

3. In the last few minutes of grilling, place cherry tomatoes on the grill to slightly char them.

4. Serve the grilled chicken topped with grilled cherry tomatoes and fresh basil leaves.

Low-FODMAP Lemon Dijon Baked Salmon

Ingredients:

• 4 salmon fillets

• Zest and juice of 1 lemon

• 2 tablespoons garlic-infused olive oil

• 2 tablespoons Dijon mustard (check for FODMAP-friendly options)

• Salt and pepper to taste

Instructions:

1. Preheat the oven to 375°F (190°C).

2. In a bowl, combine lemon zest, lemon juice, garlic-infused olive oil, Dijon mustard, salt, and pepper.

3. Place the salmon fillets in a baking dish and brush with the lemon Dijon mixture.

4. Bake for 15-20 minutes or until the salmon flakes easily.

5. Serve your lemon Dijon baked salmon with a low-FODMAP side like roasted potatoes or steamed asparagus.

Low-FODMAP Shrimp and Asparagus Pasta

Ingredients:

• 8 oz gluten-free pasta (ensure it's low-FODMAP)

• 8 oz large shrimp, peeled and deveined

• 1 cup asparagus spears, cut into bite-sized pieces

• 2 tablespoons garlic-infused olive oil

• Zest and juice of 1 lemon

• Salt and pepper to taste

• Fresh parsley for garnish

Instructions:

1. Cook gluten-free pasta according to package instructions.

2. In a skillet, heat garlic-infused olive oil over medium-high heat.

3. Add shrimp and cook until they turn pink. Add asparagus and sauté until it's tender-crisp.

4. Toss the cooked pasta, lemon zest, and lemon juice with the shrimp and asparagus. Season with salt and pepper.

5. Garnish with fresh parsley before serving.

Low-FODMAP Herb-Crusted Baked Cod

Ingredients:

• 4 cod fillets

• 2 tablespoons garlic-infused olive oil

• 2 tablespoons fresh parsley, chopped

• 2 tablespoons fresh chives, chopped

- 1/4 cup gluten-free breadcrumbs (ensure they're low-FODMAP)

- Zest of 1 lemon

- Salt and pepper to taste

Instructions:

1. Preheat the oven to 375°F (190°C).

2. In a bowl, combine garlic-infused olive oil, fresh parsley, fresh chives, gluten-free breadcrumbs, lemon zest, salt, and pepper.

3. Place the cod fillets on a baking sheet lined with parchment paper.

4. Press the herb and breadcrumb mixture onto the cod fillets. Bake for 15-20 minutes or until the cod flakes easily.

5. Serve your herb-crusted cod with a side of roasted vegetables or a quinoa salad.

Low-FODMAP Beef and Spinach Stuffed Peppers

Ingredients:

• 4 large bell peppers

• 1/2 lb ground beef

• 2 cups fresh spinach, chopped

• 1 cup cooked rice (ensure it's low-FODMAP)

• 2 tablespoons garlic-infused olive oil

• Salt and pepper to taste

Instructions:

1. Preheat the oven to 350°F (175°C). Cut the tops off the bell peppers and remove the seeds.

2. In a skillet, heat garlic-infused olive oil over medium heat. Add ground beef and cook until browned.

3. Stir in chopped spinach and cook until wilted. Add cooked rice and season with salt and pepper.

4. Stuff the bell peppers with the beef and spinach mixture. Place the stuffed peppers in a baking dish and bake for 30-35 minutes.

5. Serve your flavorful beef and spinach stuffed peppers.

Low-FODMAP Grilled Chicken Caesar Salad

Ingredients:

• 4 boneless, skinless chicken breasts

• 2 tablespoons garlic-infused olive oil

• Salt and pepper to taste

• Romaine lettuce

• Gluten-free croutons (ensure they're low-FODMAP)

• Parmesan cheese (optional)

• Low-FODMAP Caesar dressing (store-bought or homemade)

Instructions:

1. Preheat the grill to medium-high heat.

2. Season chicken breasts with salt and pepper.

3. Brush with garlic-infused olive oil and grill for 6-8 minutes per side, or until they are cooked through. Slice the grilled chicken.

4. Assemble salads with Romaine lettuce, grilled chicken slices, gluten-free croutons, and Parmesan cheese (if desired).

5. Drizzle with low-FODMAP Caesar dressing.

Low-FODMAP Lemon and Herb Grilled Swordfish

Ingredients:

• 4 swordfish steaks

• Zest and juice of 1 lemon

• 2 tablespoons garlic-infused olive oil

• 2 tablespoons fresh basil, chopped

• Salt and pepper to taste

Instructions:

1. In a bowl, combine lemon zest, lemon juice, garlic-infused olive oil, fresh basil, salt, and pepper.

2. Brush the swordfish steaks with this mixture and let them marinate for at least 30 minutes.

3. Preheat the grill to medium-high heat. Grill the swordfish for about 3-4 minutes per side, or until they are cooked through.

4. Serve with a side of roasted potatoes or a fresh green salad.

Low-FODMAP Thai Red Curry with Shrimp

Ingredients:

• 8 oz large shrimp, peeled and deveined

• 1 cup mixed low-FODMAP vegetables (e.g., bell peppers, zucchini, carrots)

• 1 can (14 oz) low-fat coconut milk

• 2 tablespoons red curry paste (check for FODMAP-friendly options)

• 2 tablespoons garlic-infused olive oil

• Salt and pepper to taste

• Fresh cilantro for garnish

• Cooked rice (ensure it's low-FODMAP)

Instructions:

1. In a large skillet, heat garlic-infused olive oil over medium heat.

2. Add shrimp and cook until they turn pink. Add mixed vegetables and stir-fry until they are tender.

3. Stir in red curry paste and sauté for a minute. Pour in low-fat coconut milk and let the mixture simmer for 10-15 minutes.

4. Season with salt and pepper.

5. Serve the Thai red curry with shrimp over cooked rice and garnish with fresh cilantro.

Low-FODMAP Grilled Lemon Garlic Shrimp

Ingredients:

• 8 oz large shrimp, peeled and deveined

• 2 tablespoons garlic-infused olive oil

• Zest and juice of 1 lemon

• 2 tablespoons fresh parsley, chopped

• Salt and pepper to taste

Instructions:

1. In a bowl, combine garlic-infused olive oil, lemon zest, lemon juice, fresh parsley, salt, and pepper.

2. Thread the shrimp onto skewers and brush them with the lemon and garlic mixture.

3. Preheat the grill to medium-high heat.

4. Grill the shrimp for about 2-3 minutes per side, or until they are pink and cooked through.

5. Serve with a side of rice or a green salad.

Low-FODMAP Quinoa and Vegetable Stir-Fry

Ingredients:

• 1 cup cooked quinoa (ensure it's low-FODMAP)

• 2 cups mixed low-FODMAP vegetables (e.g., bell peppers, carrots, snow peas)

• 2 tablespoons garlic-infused olive oil

• 2 tablespoons low-sodium soy sauce (check for FODMAP-friendly options)

• 1 tablespoon fresh ginger, minced

• Salt and pepper to taste

Instructions:

1. In a wok or skillet, heat garlic-infused olive oil over high heat.

2. Add mixed vegetables and stir-fry until they are tender. Stir in cooked quinoa and fresh ginger.

3. Drizzle with low-sodium soy sauce and season with salt and pepper.

4. Toss to combine and serve your delicious quinoa and vegetable stir-fry.

Low-FODMAP Turkey and Rice Stuffed Peppers

Ingredients:

• 4 large bell peppers

• 1/2 lb ground turkey

• 1 cup cooked rice (ensure it's low-FODMAP)

• 1/4 cup diced tomatoes

• 1/4 cup diced zucchini

• 1/4 cup diced carrots

• 2 tablespoons garlic-infused olive oil

• Salt and pepper to taste

Instructions:

1. Preheat the oven to 350°F (175°C). Cut the tops off the bell peppers and remove the seeds.

2. In a skillet, heat garlic-infused olive oil over medium heat. Add ground turkey and cook until browned.

3. Stir in diced zucchini, carrots, diced tomatoes, and cooked rice. Season with salt and pepper.

4. Stuff the bell peppers with the turkey and rice mixture. Place the stuffed peppers in a baking dish and bake for 30-35 minutes.

5. Serve your flavorful turkey and rice stuffed peppers.

Low-FODMAP Beef and Potato Skillet

Ingredients:

- 1/2 lb lean ground beef

- 2 cups diced potatoes (ensure they're low-FODMAP)

- 1 cup green beans, trimmed and cut into pieces

- 2 tablespoons garlic-infused olive oil

- Salt and pepper to taste

Instructions:

1. In a large skillet, heat garlic-infused olive oil over medium heat.

2. Add ground beef and cook until browned. Add diced potatoes and cook until they are tender and slightly crispy.

3. Stir in green beans and cook until they are tender-crisp. Season with salt and pepper.

4. Serve your hearty beef and potato skillet.

CONCLUSION

In conclusion, managing conditions like IBS, reducing stress and inflammation, and making beneficial dietary and lifestyle changes require a holistic and individualized approach. By taking a proactive role in understanding one's body and working closely with healthcare professionals, individuals can find effective strategies to improve their well-being.

For those navigating a low-FODMAP diet, the journey involves identifying dietary triggers, seeking guidance from registered dietitians, and paying attention to portion control and symptom monitoring. By understanding the specific needs of their digestive systems, individuals can create a balanced diet that supports their overall health.

In parallel, the management of stress and inflammation calls for a comprehensive approach. Incorporating stress-reduction techniques, engaging in regular physical activity, and cultivating a support network are vital components of a healthy lifestyle. By embracing these changes, individuals can enhance their emotional well-being and manage stress, ultimately reducing the impact of inflammation on their health.

Recognizing that dietary choices can have a profound impact on digestive health and stress levels, incorporating foods with calming effects on the digestive system can be beneficial. These foods, along with portion control and an understanding of one's triggers, can provide a valuable tool in the management of IBS and overall well-being.

The journey towards better health is a continuous one. It requires patience, self-awareness, and adaptability. By implementing the strategies discussed and seeking professional guidance, individuals can take proactive steps toward improving their quality of life and effectively managing their health challenges.

www.ingramcontent.com/pod-product-compliance
Lightning Source LLC
Chambersburg PA
CBHW070940260726
48661CB00003B/1057